THAI
MASSAGE
DISSECTED

Praise for *Thai Massage Dissected*

Natasha set out to provide a comprehensive guide to the practice of Thai massage and has achieved much more. Combining Natasha's wealth of direct tuition from masters of both Thai bodywork and anatomical dissections, Thai Massage Dissected seamlessly blends the two worlds to give a comprehensive and grounded overview of the multi-faceted therapy.

This book is about connections – from anatomical to spiritual, between client and therapist, from practice to expertise. The full-body approach, so beautifully illustrated throughout Thai Massage Dissected, will help you put your client back together.

James Earls
MSc, author of *Born to Walk* and
Understanding the Human Foot
www.borntomove.com

My first recommendation for yoga teachers and therapists wanting to develop their touch and understanding of applied body mechanics has always been to study Thai massage. To go even deeper, my follow-up suggestion is to do a dissection course, as there is nothing like it to witness the beauty and sacredness of our inner world. Natasha has managed here to share her amazing knowledge and wisdom within an accessible book that will likely become a classic to anyone wanting a deeper glimpse into the human form. My third and final piece of advice is to delve into this volume – your clients and students will surely thank you for it.

Raphan Kebe
Founder of Space & Flow Yoga™ and host of the
'Talking, Teaching & Flow' podcast

Natasha has created a beautiful, elegant and comprehensive book which will be essential to anyone interested in or practicing Thai massage.

Thai Massage Dissected gives the reader the opportunity to deepen their understanding of this ancient practice through the author's teachings and findings. There is not a more in-depth book available. Natasha's passion, knowledge and research into her subject are clearly present throughout the book. She brings her personal insights to the practice, making it accessible and modern but without losing touch or respect for the history. Reading this book felt like taking a spiritual journey.

Jeannie Di Bon
Movement therapist, author of
Pilates Without Tears and
Hypermobility Without Tears. Host of
'Finding Your Range' podcast
www.jeanniedibon.com

This is an incredibly exciting resource for practitioners across the world. Within, you'll find the meeting place of more recent body-knowledge and the older sciences/medicines of a traditional practice. Natasha also makes some important corrections to common misinformation in the field, and builds you an essential base of Thai medical theory upon which you may formulate a practice. Teachers and practitioners alike would do well to leverage this powerful educational resource for enhancing understanding, clarity in, and execution of this therapy we all hold so dearly.

Drew Hume
Thai Massage teacher navina.ca

I am so delighted to see this book out in the world! Natasha is a gifted healer and teacher who has a deep knowledge of this therapeutic tradition and it is really showcased in this book. Thai Massage Dissected is a practical and comprehensive guide to Thai massage. Natasha has taken all her years of practice and experience and gifted it to us in this beautiful book!

Jonelle Lewis
Yoga teacher, educator and mentor.
Co-founder of the Radical Darshan
Yoga School

THAI MASSAGE DISSECTED

NATASHA DE GRUNWALD

FOREWORD BY
GIL HEDLEY

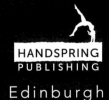

HANDSPRING
PUBLISHING

Edinburgh

HANDSPRING PUBLISHING LIMITED
The Old Manse, Fountainhall,
Pencaitland, East Lothian
EH34 5EY, Scotland
Tel: +44 1875 341 859
Website: www.handspringpublishing.com

First published 2021 in the United Kingdom by Handspring Publishing Limited
Copyright © Handspring Publishing Limited 2021

ISBN 978-1-913426-11-8
ISBN (Kindle eBook) 978-1-913426-12-5

British Library Cataloguing in Publication Data
A catalogue record for this book is available from the British Library
Library of Congress Cataloguing in Publication Data
A catalog record for this book is available from the Library of Congress

Commissioning Editor Sarena Wolfaard
Project Manager Morven Dean
Copyeditor Wendy Lee
Designer Kirsteen Wright
Illustrator Rebecca Connor
Photographer Katya de Grunwald
Model Anoushka de Grunwald Crépaud
Indexer Aptara, India
Typesetter Ditech, India
Printer Finidr, Czech Republic

The
Publisher's
policy is to use
paper manufactured
from sustainable forests

Contents

Contents

About the Author

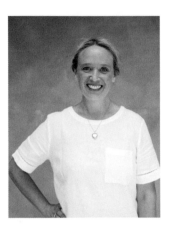

Natasha de Grunwald first studied Thai Massage in 1990 in Thailand and has returned there to continue her studies more than 16 times. She has travelled extensively, learning from teachers across the globe from New Zealand to New York to Serbia. Her pursuit for knowledge has led her to the Burmese borders to research with village midwives, to training with a Reusi (the Thai equivalent of a Shaman), and into a cadaver lab many times.

Having had a busy private practice since 1990, and having worked at Great Ormond Street Hospital at the very beginning of her career, throwing herself in at the deep end by massaging women whose young children were dying from AIDS, Natasha has always been a practitioner with great insight and a passion to transform lives through touch.

In 2005 she opened London Institute of Thai Yoga Massage with a commitment to raising the standards and putting Thai bodywork on the map as a reputable physical therapy. She has since trained thousands of people from around the world and continues to do so, offering the UK's only 300-hour programme and as the only UK teacher of therapeutic Thai massage and bodywork.

Foreword by Gil Hedley

Like the astronauts who navigate outer space, the Somanaut navigates the inner space of the human form. In so doing, she discovers her own inner nature as well. Natasha de Grunwald is a genuine Somanaut! I can personally testify to her status as such, having spent many weeks in the lab with her discovering the actual territory of the human body, the land that the maps of the anatomy books only vaguely point towards. She is a committed explorer of inner space. Natasha's enthusiasm for learning is unbridled, and her commitment to challenging her own perceptions is a credit to her as a teacher. She delights in having her perspectives turned upside down, so much the better for seeing things anew. She does not accept the status quo of her knowledge as complete but returns to the table again and again to expand her perceptions for herself and, by extension, for her students of Thai massage.

One of the great benefits of delving so far into dissection is that one develops a kind of "X-ray vision" through this type of hands-on study that is hard to come by otherwise. Those who dissect as de Grunwald has are afforded the ability to see what they touch, to visualize more accurately their patients'/clients' anatomical particularities and so serve them better. Her many times repeated experience also enables her to convey to her students a sense of human anatomy from a depth that could never be achieved from mere book study. I respect Natasha for repeatedly challenging herself to return to the lab, a place not for the faint of heart, in her quest for excellence in her practice and teaching.

It also takes a lot of courage to teach and write while knowing your knowledge is incomplete and your understanding and perceptions are still growing. Anyone who has ever dared to teach and write knows what I am talking about. Most medical students have heard one of their professors quip that "Half of what we teach you is wrong ... and we don't know which half!" In the Thai tradition, like many other ancient systems, there is some expectation that you might teach only once you "know it all." Anything less might be considered dangerous or irresponsible at best. With this, there may be an assumption that a teacher's knowledge can be complete, and all principles at some point mastered.

While I deeply respect this tradition, I do not subscribe to this particular principle myself. I originally started teaching dissection with only about a four-day head start on my course participants in terms of lab experience – cheeky, I admit. But I did know how to learn, and to lead with my own excitement for discovery, and I continue to do so. Knowledge and depth are infinite, and you will surely expire before you know it all! So, from this non-traditional perspective, at some point you pluck up the courage to share what you know. This is precisely what de Grunwald has done here in the chapters that follow. She has done this in the service of humanity, with deep humility, conscious that what she conveys will always be partial and incomplete, particularly in the face of so vast a subject. But even so, it will be enough for those of you who study along with her, for now. There are sufficient gems between the cover of this book to keep you mining them for a good while. And as time passes, the base of your understanding will continue to grow with hers, just as it did before she dared to teach and write.

The key is to be up-front with the partial nature of all knowledge, and to bear willingly the responsibility to improve relentlessly and to develop one's understanding and its applications. Students bear this responsibility too, and it is incumbent on the teacher to lead in this forward movement. Natasha de Grunwald is just such a courageous and responsible practitioner and teacher. She is genuinely humbled and filled with wonder by the vast world of the human body, so many mysteries of which remain beyond our understanding still. For her, teaching and writing are as much a process of discovery and exploration as dissection, all learning processes. She does not need to "know it all" in order to inculcate respect and appreciation for the body, or to generate excitement for learning among her students, as well as to convey with heart everything she has to offer from her several decades of invaluable experience.

In what follows, de Grunwald applies that substantial experience with the Thai massage and medical traditions to challenge some of their more rote aspects. She brings it forward, alive and growing, right along with her. I appreciate her willingness to share in this way. Her gentle approach and her ability to tailor the techniques are a testament to her respect not only for the Thai tradition, but for the unique needs of each person she serves. For de Grunwald, her own healing journey serves as a cautionary tale to would-be, as well as experienced, practitioners to respect the body, listen to its whispers, study its complexities and deliver what a person needs, as opposed to a stock treatment. Enjoy the exploration: you are fortunate to have come upon this sage guide.

Gil Hedley, Ph.D.

Melbourne, Florida, USA

February 2021

Preface

My inspiration for writing this book was kindled many years ago when I began searching for, and then researching, Thai medicine.

I had been frustrated for a long time, as I was reading Thai massage books which all seemed to present sequences of techniques and stretches but were lacking in theory. Most of what I could find seemed to stem from the Chinese or Ayurvedic systems but it was Thai theory I was seeking. I wanted to be able to work therapeutically with clients and knew that to have more depth in my work there had to be more options than learning about stretching.

I excitedly devoured the tiny amount of literature I could find written in English on Thai medicine and massage. Increasingly, my students were also asking me for reading recommendations. I was generally pointing them to a couple of books at best.

If ancient, Eastern knowledge intrigues you and you also like anatomy, I think you will be pleasantly surprised when you discover therapeutic Thai bodywork and begin looking at the body through a completely different lens.

In my thirty years as a practitioner, teacher, and researcher, this modality is the richest and most diverse I have found. It contains components of all other modalities within it. It spans from visceral manipulation to deep joint traction, from applied stretching to subtle touch and esoteric techniques, from myofascial release to work with neuro-vascular bundles. Thai bodywork practitioners can therefore place themselves easily alongside all other physical therapy practices, if they have learned from the traditional model which teaches Thai anatomy and medical theory.

The scope for therapeutic work (which is also easy on the practitioner's body) makes it very magnetic and explains why practitioners of other modalities want to implement it in their work.

In recent years, I have trained a growing number of sports massage practitioners, physiotherapists, osteopaths, and yoga teachers, and the results they achieve are incredible.

In the Western world, Thai massage is mainly known as a relaxing treatment that involves pressing, thumbing, and stretching throughout a two-hour session. But from the therapeutic angle, relaxation is not the primary goal. There are countless different techniques using hands or tools, such as cupping therapy, scarf work, spoon scraping, and subtle therapies that are similar to cranio-sacral work, which reset the nervous system. This book explores these lesser-known traditional and therapeutic approaches so that Thai physical therapy can be put on the map as the effective, diverse, healing modality that it is, rich in Thai medical theory.

The writing of this book comes from my desire to impart the knowledge and experience I have of teaching and implementing Thai bodywork and working closely with people, and what that work is like in practice, while ensuring that, to the best of my ability, I acknowledge the lineage of Thai medicine that I study, teach, and practice.

My massage is predominantly carried out in the Western world and involves working closely with people here. I study and observe how they move and function, along with the obvious links and interconnectivity between mental and emotional health, the soul and the physical body.

The benefits of my time spent dissecting cadavers in a lab took me to new levels of learning and understanding, both personally and professionally, and gave me a profound curiosity about the miracle of life, human form and behavior, and the internal universe. This area of my work keeps me questioning. The insights gained from the experience assist me in having a wide perspective to help me work with the many complex layers of the whole person, and to share this knowledge with students who train with me or read this book.

My studies in Thai medicine are an on-going journey, requiring patience and dedication, and even after thirty years I know there is always much more to learn. So I am a teacher, but always a student. There are lists to learn off by heart, the precise order of items on these lists being important and symbolic, steeped in Buddhism and traditional Thai culture. Each aspect of knowledge involves a lot of thought and comprehension to allow for deeper study. The theory is not something that can be learned quickly; it is not for the impatient. For those of us in the West who cannot live in Thailand and who do not speak the language there will always be gaps in the ancient knowledge, but despite this, the efficacy of this lens is unmistakable.

I realized that if I waited until I had acquired all the knowledge of Thai medical theory or the body, or had seen every possible condition through all lenses and somehow found a way to put it all into words, the book would never be written and I would be an old woman.

This book comes from years of teaching and from noticing what students need, where they get stuck, and the questions I hear them ask over and over again about putting the theory into practice and making a success of what they do. It is intended as a resource for students and practitioners from all modalities,

from which they may gain insights. It is not intended to be a definitive guide to Thai medical theory or anatomy, but I hope the insights I have gained over nearly three decades will help you in your practice as it evolves and your knowledge deepens. For those beginners who want to learn how to massage the body with ease and without tiring, this will be also be invaluable reading. There are many techniques that are almost unbelievable, as they are so effective but do not require the practitioner to strain their own body.

The Thai medicine lineage in which I teach, practice, and study is a precious heritage, very much in danger of being lost forever.

A teacher said to me that there are three things that make a living tradition:

- a vast body of knowledge written in ancient texts as a reference

- a need for a teacher to give instruction, demonstrate, and preserve the traditions and knowledge

- people practicing the art.

This teacher is a doctor and a Reusi (the Thai equivalent of a Yogi or Shaman) who has studied all five roots of Thai medicine, and it is because of this vast knowledge and his being a devout Buddhist and Reusi that he is very well respected in Thailand. He has teachers who are village doctors, spirit doctors, herbalists, and monks, and who have entrusted him with traditional knowledge which he is dedicated to preserving and which he and other teachers have shared with me.

This book is written with the information that I currently hold, informed by the opinions I presently have, acknowledging that I still have so much more to learn (thankfully) and that as I grow so will the body of knowledge that I am able to share. My opinions are likely to evolve as I go deeper into the medicine and my perspective might shift, because that is the nature of being a life-long student. Throughout this book I have included knowledge that comes from my own observations, studies, and clinical practice spanning thirty years, some of which do not form part of Thai medicine.

I hope this book inspires others to study the body, especially through dissection, and to keep an open and forward-thinking mind in their clinical observations when working with clients.

I hope it leads to your own questioning, reflecting, and developing an inquisitive mind, as this is what promotes growth.

Most importantly, I hope it inspires more people to understand the true power of therapeutic touch, to be able to reach out to those in the community who are lacking physical connection, and to use the many tools a Thai practitioner has available to help people feel at ease in their body.

Thai and Lanna medicine

Before we delve in, this seems like an appropriate time for a brief mention of the history and distortion related to this modality in years gone by.

The approach you will find in this book is one of medical massage using diagnostics, theory, and therapeutic treatment-oriented outcomes, in line with traditional medicine. Most of the information I share here comes from Lanna medicine or local medicine practitioners.

However, the style of Thai massage most commonly practiced throughout the world is a standardized system that has been promoted by the Ministry of Health in Thailand. This version mixes Ayurvedic and Western philosophies into the medicine while also gathering information from old practitioners. Once all of this knowledge is assembled, it is then watered down, many traditional aspects being either completely left out or changed to fit the Western medicine model.

Local medicine, or "village medicine" as it is often known, is based on a variety of practices which come from local practitioners and documented texts. There are many more variants in the "local doctor/medicine" category, and many more traditional practices are found.

Lanna medicine comes from the Lanna people, who settled in Northern Thailand many centuries ago. They do not consider themselves as Thai at all, but see themselves as belonging to a separate ethnicity. Their own system of medicine is the best-preserved traditional medicine of Thailand, with medical Lanna texts that date back to the thirteenth century. The Lanna people also have their own specialized medical practices, such as Tok Sên, cupping, and scraping, which have become part of Thai medicine.

Natasha de Grunwald

London, UK

March 2021

Acknowledgments

With thanks to:

Anoushka de Grunwald Crépaud

Michael Jenkins

Gil Hedley

Tevijo Yogi

Nephyr Jacobsen

Rachel Fettiplace

Hope Nicholson

Kathryn Entwistle

Katya de Grunwald

David Crépaud

Suzy Ashworth

Pierce Salguero

Lise Flora Waugh

Danko La Radic

Thai/Lanna medicine community and all the teachers in Thailand, past and present

All students who have trained with me over the years, and from whom I have learned so much.

Donors

I would like to give special thanks to all the donors and their families. The donors have been prominent teachers in my life, whom I never met when they were alive but who have taught me so much. They had the foresight to bequeath their bodies to science and I was a recipient of their parting gift. I am eternally grateful to these wise souls, and I know it is from their generosity that I am able to teach and practice with real insight into human form.

Introduction

I was born six days after my maternal grandmother died, and because of this I was almost named Phoenicia, as in the phoenix rising, symbolizing resurrection, new life, transformation. My mother, ahead of her time in her thinking, always said to me that she thinks I felt her pain when I was in utero, and has often suggested to me that this is why I am an empath, highly aware of and sensitive to other people's energy, mood, and unspoken communications, just as I would have been to hers in the womb.

One thing is for sure: for my whole life I have been observing people and the world around me. I know this because I distinctly remember sitting on my nursery school teacher's big, cozy, green chair, day after day, watching all the children playing. I would sit there for long periods, rarely getting up to join in. I remember being immersed in watching, taking it all in, thumb in mouth.

I was able to see so many things as I sat there: interactions and dynamics between the other children, changes in energy in the room. I could see the teacher's frustration building up.

Of course, I had no words for this, but I remember the imagery and sensations in my body so vividly. This really was the start of my interest in human behavior, one that has continued to grow to this present day and has certainly shaped me as a teacher and practitioner, giving me an acute awareness and an ability to sense non-verbal, energetic shifts and communications strongly.

Aspects of my childhood years were troubled. There was a lot of conflict and disharmony at home; my dad left and my stepmother had mental health issues which affected the whole family in indescribable ways. My mum was involved in a counseling community and I grew up with people coming to the house for therapy. My upbringing shaped me, and on the positive side it taught me about suffering, healing, and personal growth from a young age, and gave me a passion and vision to help others transform their lives and reach their full potential, no matter what barriers were in their way.

I started teaching very young: I was only eleven years old when I led a class for young people in the counseling community that my mum was involved in (this mostly consisted of dancing, moving, and using our voices to shout out what feelings we were experiencing, and then laughing a lot).

I was fourteen when my boyfriend knocked out my two front teeth. Preceding and following that, there had been a flood of violent physical and emotional abuse from him. I was terrified all the time. I was thin, skeletal. My periods stopped. Life was miserable and confusing; I was disconnected from my peers and isolated, too ashamed to tell anyone. I became so far removed from myself that I barely gave myself a thought. I was in a highly anxious state, not functioning and in a state of trauma, yet back then, of course, I did not realize this.

For the next few years I struggled. I was completely lost and traumatized, so I tried to escape by taking drugs and moving through the world in a fog.

I reached a stage where my body was numb. I was totally disconnected from it. I saw a counselor, who massaged my feet as I talked with her. I saw an acupuncturist because I literally could not feel my body – I could scratch an itch on my arm and see I was scratching it but I could not feel anything. My liver was inflamed and my cheeks were sunken.

Yet, thankfully, I had wonderful support from a family friend, whom I saw as my therapist and who constantly reminded me of the person she saw beneath the veil that I had created. From this, I found a spark of life in me. There was also an unconscious drive: small seeds had been planted that illuminated another way for me to go. I made a choice and started to form a new path for myself.

In 1989, aged eighteen, l took an aromatherapy and holistic massage course, but soon realized that rubbing some oil around on someone's skin was not going to satisfy my desire really to help people at a deep level. I must have subconsciously known that it would not have been enough to help me heal either. So, I left everything behind and went to Thailand with a friend, in search of traditional Thai massage.

It was then that I started finding myself. I experienced hope, freedom, and lightness again. There is a vitality in Thailand, and a culture so completely different to what I knew. This, combined with being massaged deeply almost every day, meant I started to connect to my body again. The deep work was incredibly healing, as it seemed to wake me up to myself. I felt it lit me back up and connected the dots of my physical, emotional, and spiritual self, repairing my central nervous system from the suffering and effects of drug taking.

After one particular massage that I received within the quiet of temple grounds (where I later trained; see photo at right), I sat for a long time in a strange state that I could not recognize. My body felt like jelly; I felt calm, content, slow, grounded, with liquid freedom in my tissues. (I can describe these feelings now, as I know them well, but at the time I just sat, unable to move or speak for two hours.) I knew that something powerful had happened.

As I sat there in a kind of trance, I felt life and nourishment running back through my body; I had hope.

With hindsight, I can see this was another massive turning point. It was a time which turned the experience of my body into a positive one again, and I knew at that point that Thai massage would be a large part of my life. I had no idea then that, thirty years later, I would be teaching this modality, having researched and studied it for all these years, curious to understand what had created the powerful transformation.

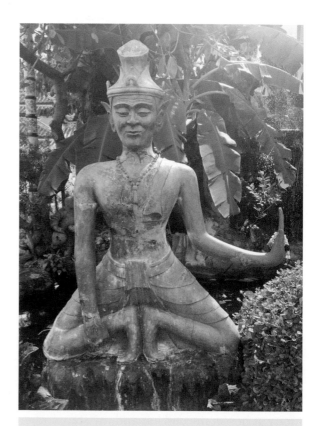

Reusi statue in the grounds of a temple in central Bangkok, where I first trained.

The regular strong massages touched me; they helped me find myself again and gave me a new sense of myself at a very deep level. The strong effect that deep, intentional, therapeutic touch can trigger in the body is something that continues to inspire me and makes me ever-curious. What does it mean to be touched like this? What happens when we are lacking in physical touch? What happens when we do not have physical, emotional, and spiritual support? How is it that touch can help us notice ourselves at a deep level? Why do emotions come up when the body is worked on? How can something as simple as touch awaken our soul?

Part of the reason I tell this story is that it was the intense and therapeutic work on my body that produced this strong effect. However, there were many years during which I gave Thai massage using a gentler, sequence-based approach. It was very relaxing but ultimately it was a generic treatment, heavy on the stretches and without any real theory attached to it. There was a noticeable lack of access to teachers and knowledge at this time, so I was giving treatments with three standard techniques (palming, thumbing, and stretching). No matter how hard I tried, I could not find theory that was Thai. I kept bumping up against Chinese and yoga philosophy and it did not quite fit. The lack of depth of knowledge was holding back my practice from helping people reach the next level in their health and wellbeing, and my frustration started increasing rapidly. There was a key component missing and I went on a mission to find it.

What I discovered is that when Thai massage is approached through the lens of Thai medical theory, it is an extremely therapeutic modality, a physical therapy that could be compared to, and has elements of, **cranio-sacral** therapy, **Rolfing**, physiotherapy, sports massage, myofascial release, and osteopathy. It has an extremely broad scope for healing, encompassing the physical, spiritual, energetic, and emotional facets of one's being.

Despite the reputation for being deep physical work, there are also subtle and gentle touch techniques for working on the body. These fascinate me, as light touch techniques are often the most effective, giving space for the soul to respond without force or overkill of input. The recipient goes into a receptive state of acceptance. This is highly creative and healing, as the mind ultimately has the most powerful effect on the physical body.

At the very beginning of my career, I worked for a charity, run by nuns, for women with HIV/AIDS. Every week for ten years, from the age of nineteen, I would massage these women who had lived through atrocities in Africa. Some of them also had very sick children, and part of my work was to massage the mothers at Great Ormond Street Hospital in London where they were at their children's bedside, or in other central London hospitals where they themselves were dying. This important work shaped my career. It was not the "normal" start for such a young massage therapist. The professional relationships I had with these women, the support I was able to give them and their families, was profound, for them and for me.

When I first decided to enroll on a dissection course, I had no idea what would happen. But I knew it was the right next step for me: I really wanted to learn more about the body. I was both excited and terrified, a good sign that it was going to be the thing to take me forwards.

Introduction

In the lead-up to the first day, when I was on the precipice of something very new (an experience only for the brave), I was dreaming of the dead, seeing cadavers in my sleep – many souls visited me in those nights.

Within six days of being in the lab, my mind had been blown open. This course was not just learning about the body, it was like seeing inner space. My state of consciousness altered and my view of the body was transformed. My teacher, Gil Hedley, had led me to a new universe which could be discovered in depth, and my curiosity had no limits.

By the last day of the dissection, I knew I had leaped into a completely new space, one from which there was no return. In those first six days, my perspective on life really changed forever: personally, professionally, spiritually, experientially. The experience is so profound that I have returned for many more dissection courses since.

I believe the biggest leaps of faith are the ones that make us feel most alive and connected to our own source. The sheer terror and excitement of being far out of a comfort zone are always the best experiences and take those that are willing to a place of expansion.

Thai bodywork and manual therapy is a vehicle for change. It changes the lives of the recipients seeking healing but, most interestingly, it changes the lives of the practitioners too.

As I go deeper into my teachings and my training school expands, I realize I can no longer teach physical therapy without teaching about the soul, the mind, and the emotional components that make us human. Learning about touch inevitably becomes a journey of self-growth and self-awareness, one in which the practitioner can mirror and lead clients on their own path.

PART 1

The Experience

1 The Somatic Experience

When it comes to healing therapies, there really is nothing better than therapeutic Thai bodywork.

My observations of what happens during a Thai massage are where this book begins. Thai bodywork is not like any other modality — or more precisely, it is like many modalities all rolled into one and then seen through a completely different lens. Its effects and the experience are profound. This is not superficial bodywork by any stretch of the imagination; it has a long history of incredible efficacy.

People often inaccurately believe that giving Thai massage must be really hard work or at least fairly tiring. This could not be further from the truth, but it comes from the experience of the client who is lying on a floor mat being massaged, often with their eyes closed, and stems from the fact that the pressure, stretches, and range of techniques feel strangely different and deeply effective; they really do hit that "sweet spot." And to be honest, it *is* very different to other modalities. The Thai practitioner is not actually working hard at all, but uses gravity, movement, and leaning, which, if applied correctly and with enough practice, are deceptively easy on the therapist's own body. This is bodywork for practitioners who

care deeply about giving transformative treatments, but without exhausting themselves in the process.

Thai massage *is* unusual, in that it is powerful and fulfilling for *both* participants. Many other styles of manual therapy leave the practitioner exhausted or heading for burn-out. Repetitive strain injuries are commonplace. Yet Thai bodywork leaves both practitioner and recipient in a state of heightened awareness, openness, and relaxation. The practitioner is simultaneously giving and receiving.

The recipient is participating in the treatment by noticing themselves, often at a deep level, their proprioception dial turned up (see Chapter 2 for more on this term). The provider is also taking note of their own body with heightened awareness *and* attention to how it is interacting with the recipient's body; there is a strong **symbiotic** relationship formed in the shared experience.

Practitioners use a broader perspective when giving Thai massage. They are not concentrating on the muscle and soft tissue layer, but are intentionally treating deeper layers, and the physiology of the body.

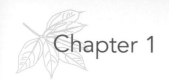
For recipients, this leads to a deepening of their internal viewpoint, and creates a much more profound experience and **awakeness** (it wakes people up to themselves).

The Thai practitioner effortlessly performs techniques that encourage the soft tissue structure to adjust, allowing them to go deeper into the body and stimulate the **Sên**. Sên is the collective term for all pathways of movement in the body: the neuro-vascular bundles, lymphatic system, tendons, and ligaments (see Chapter 10 for more on this).

The adjustment to the soft tissue stimulates a change in the general function of the body and can be seen moving through the body-wide chain of joints or muscles. The soft tissue layer is nerve-rich. With the practitioner consistently applying manual therapy techniques to the **fascia** and deeper Sên, it directly impacts all other systems in the body as Wind element (movement) is activated along the pathways.

Side note: Wind is the element that is synonymous with movement (more about this later in Chapter 3). But for now, if you read "Wind," know that it means movement.

Directly stimulating the **channels** in the body creates a whole-body, physiological change as the Sên that lie beneath them become less obstructed. For example, the nerves can move more easily in their fascial casing, resulting in an increase in communication along neural pathways. The implication of a nerve no longer being pressed on by the surrounding tissue

has an impact that ranges from the physical to the emotional. If this tiny neural structure has greater freedom to enjoy being unrestricted, the soul is eventually allowed to express itself.

In Thai bodywork the therapist systematically addresses the layers of the body, making sure that each one is taken care of before the next is worked on. This is a gentle, safe, and effective way of accessing the deeper layers of the body, in such a way that the body does not resist the touch or find it painful in a non-therapeutic or unpleasant way. When cared for properly, each layer softens so that the practitioner's touch can sink in deeper without force. There are times when only the skin and second layer can be worked on, when tissue is so bound up that it needs time to soften and become more fluid. Rushing this phase of a treatment is not productive or effective, and is likely to inhibit the powerful therapeutic response.

"Speed is the enemy of sensitivity; move at or below the rate of tissue melting."

Thomas Myers, 2009

The Recipient's Experience

The direct application of touch to the skin stimulates the **somatosensory system** (which is part of the sensory nervous system) and sends impulses to the brain via the spinal cord. A light touch can travel very quickly along the nerve tree (Fig. 1.1) in the body, the branches of which are far-reaching.

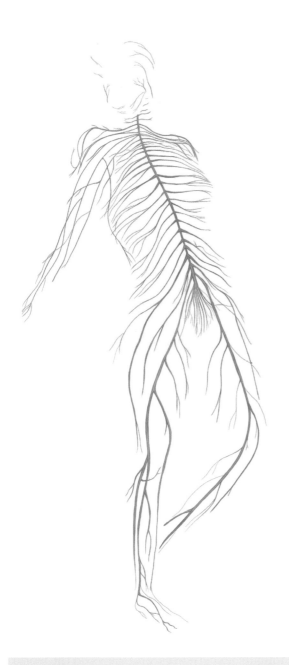

Fig. 1.1
Nerve tree.

Techniques such as rubbing, performed to warm the skin layer, can be vigorous yet soothing, and the whole body responds as reassuring waves of warmth ripple through it. Techniques that address the second layer (soft tissue, muscles, and fascia) encourage the fibers to release some of their tension and held memory. The soul softens, the tissues hydrate. The touch itself generates a deepened sensory experience of the perception of oneself. Fluids are replenished and there is an exchange of nutrients.

The applied stretches stimulate Wind element, from the physical movement of that limb to the stimulation of underlying nerves embedded in the tissue, causing many proprioceptive awakenings. Vibration, traction, and range of motion are applied to the bone layer, which influence the fascia and chain of joints that stack above and below, from feet to head. **Lymph nodes** are massaged, which has a direct impact on lymphatic flow, encouraging a cleansing of waste and toxins from the body. The **viscera** and internal organs are massaged to promote their optimum function, and the breath deepens. The **tentorium cerebelli**, a membrane in the cerebellum of the brain, moves as the limbs are moved.

Massage techniques such as **"plucking"** around the neck at the **sternocleidomastoid**

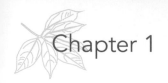

stimulate the **vagus nerve** that meanders down through the body to the internal organs, directly influencing them and the **parasympathetic** nervous system (while the **enteric** nervous system is influencing the vagus nerve in a reciprocal arrangement). While massaging this area, the therapist gains an awareness of the connections and fascial continuities that reach up to the cranium (**galea aponeurotica**) and down to the front of the hips (anterior superior iliac spine), covering the distance between and beyond. Applying touch to the anterior neck area can help to relieve hip pain or assist a deeper breath to the diaphragm or belly.

Often, after receiving Thai massage, clients have a look of childlike wonder on their face, as if they have just been part of an incredible magic show. What they seem to be experiencing is encountering their body in a whole new and different way. Their perception of themselves has altered. They have been taken through a sequence of movements that they may never have thought possible of their own body. They have experienced profound and therapeutic touch that has awakened deeper aspects of themselves. They have had a treatment that not only works on the muscle layer of the body but has focused on physiology: nerves have been stimulated, the lymphatic system has been worked on, the viscera have been massaged, and joints have been mobilized.

When the physical body and the soul feel relief from pain, tension, and stress, a general sense of wellbeing, self-connection, and restored equilibrium is created. Thai massage makes the client relaxed but energized, an unusual combination. Recipients may also mention a feeling of electricity and warmth running through them, which is due to improved blood circulation and hydration, along with a stronger body awareness as the nerves wake up. Other effects that are frequently reported are a feeling of greater freedom in the body, as well as postural improvements, injury rehabilitation, reduced pain, greater vitality, and a better connection to an interoceptive experience.

As the body releases deep-held tension, it is common for emotions to come to the surface and also to be released. This is a clear example of how working on the physical body (Earth and Water) dispels stagnation. As Wind element moves through the body and mind, it affects the internal chemistry, so often there is a wave of heat (Fire element) that rushes through the system before the emotional release. Crying is the body's intelligent and effective way of freeing stress chemicals, literally flushing them out through tears. These tears can clear the way for clearer thought patterns and help the recipient feel much better.

The Practitioner's Experience

Performing acts of kindness, demonstrating compassion, creating connection, and simply touching another person (one of the most primal ways of communicating) are all reasons why the practitioner will truly benefit from giving the massage.

When you are working as a practitioner, there may be times that you get into discussions with clients about their lives, private thoughts, experiences, and views on the world. This can come into the consultation or the treatment: as people relax, they often want to talk; or if the session is painful, talking can be a good distraction. The narrative, and having a safe space for communication, are essential aspects of therapeutic work.

Massage takes a focus and attention to detail that requires you to be very aware in the moment of *exactly* what is happening. Every touch or tool is applied accurately with detailed and tailored work. The benefits are huge for the giver. When the mind is kept focused on one thing alone, the process resembles a meditation, which has a positive effect on mood, happiness, and pain levels.

"It appears people who are better able to control their attention are also better able to control their pain."

Todd Hargrove, 2014

During the session, **kinetic** energy (the energy of movement) is engaged when the stretches, range of motion, beating, traction, and vibration are performed. These movements are either fluid or dynamic, and the practitioner constantly moves into a variety of postures while carrying them out. This movement is beneficial, keeping the practitioner agile and flexible in their own body.

The practitioner pays attention to the sensation of touch that they are receiving while giving the massage because this is a two-way street: in applying touch, there is immediate and vital feedback.

There are times when the practitioner applies techniques that are long holds; there is no movement at all, and at these points there is intense awareness, similar to a meditative practice with heightened, intentional focus.

"Intricate energy interactions occur between nearby individuals even if they are not in physical contact. Seeing and talking with another person are energetic interactions, involving light and sound vibrations … add therapeutic touch to the equation and whole new dimensions of subtle but measurable exchanges are bought into play."

James L. Oschman, 2000

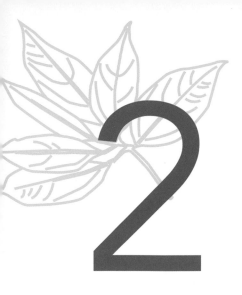

2 Proprioception, Interoception, and Touch Perception

Proprioception is "the awareness of body position in space" (oxfordreference.com). **Interoception** is "sensitivity to stimuli originating inside of the body" (collinsdictionary.com).

In this chapter I am encouraging you to think about proprioception, interoception, and **touch receptors** while you work with individual clients, as it will heighten your ability to create effective and profound treatments for them while connecting you more to your own experience of these.

Proprioception

Yoga teacher Jill Miller describes proprioception as:

"Your body's sense of itself; your inner GPS system. The ability to sense the position, location, orientation and movement of your body and its parts."

Jill Miller, 2014

Proprioception is often written about as a self-awareness concept, yet in Thai massage there are two people involved in the treatment and so the practitioner needs to have a strong awareness of their own body, as well as that of the recipient. Similarly, the recipient will have a reciprocal awareness of the practitioner's body, as it is interlinked with their own orientation.

Movement plays a key role in Thai massage, often much more so than in any other modality. It is the focus in many forms throughout a session. Passive movement (range of motion, vibration, stretching, and traction) is carried out on the recipient's body, which is moved into various postures, and which may be moved or asked to move from supine to prone to seated or side-lying in a session. Additionally, there is the movement of the practitioner to consider, who frequently moves around while performing the massage. This movement is informed by a proprioceptive self-awareness, and by reflection of the practitioner on how they are moving through space around the recipient.

In a treatment there are many moments of stillness during long, slow, deep compressions or the performance of subtle **Wind Gate** work. These require the practitioner to be completely present and to have great focus on their own body and that of the recipient, so that the work can be targeted and effective. There are other times when therapists use the foot, elbow, or

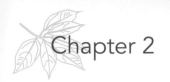
shin to carry out the treatment, and so they must have good proprioception to be able to apply these effectively and safely.

The space created when having a massage, and especially with the deeply healing aspect of Thai massage, often invokes inward meditation (interoception) and a proprioceptive exploration for both participants. The practitioner is exploring how the recipient's body can be moved through space and the recipient is experiencing their own body being moved. From this, we can see that proprioception and interoception become core components of the session.

"Movement is a relative concept – it only exists in relation to something else."

Donna Finando, 2005

Proprioception stems from the external stimuli arising from body position, movement, and touch. The practitioner needs to have acute awareness of their own body throughout the session, and of the movements performed on the client.

Proprioception is communicated via the skin and the superficial and deep fascia. These components of the second layer (categorized in Thai medicine as an Earth element body part) are rich in nerve endings while also being highly intelligent structures that have waves and force conducted through them while in motion. The nerve endings are a continuation of the central nervous system, and capillaries a continuation of the heart. Fascia is a sensory organ and a "sensory signaling feedback system" (Joanne Avison, 2015).

What this means is that there is a two-way communication system going on. The practitioner is using the Earth element of their body to give the massage, and their body functions as a natural fascial antenna that picks up and sends out information. Alongside this, the antenna of the recipient's body is doing the same (Fig. 2.1).

Interoception

Interoception is the internal perception we have of ourselves, which provides the foundation for sensory feelings and greater self-awareness. It is a communication system between the body and all its internal physiological states – a two-way highway. Heartbeat, breathing, hunger, emotional awareness, and an individual's response to stress are among many physiological, non-conscious states we can experience in response to internal stimuli, and all are classified as interoception. Interoception can be seen as a precursor to, and even a blueprint for, emotional response.

It is very common these days, with many people operating on autopilot and often being highly stressed, for us to lose touch with how we are at a core level. We become numb to our internal experiences and disconnected from ourselves. We are often so heavily embroiled in "doing and reacting" but lack the connection to ourselves that is needed for general health and wellbeing, and this becomes a negative cycle. This disconnect often has a very damaging and serious impact on physical and mental health. If internal perception (interoception) were given greater importance, a lot of suffering could be avoided.

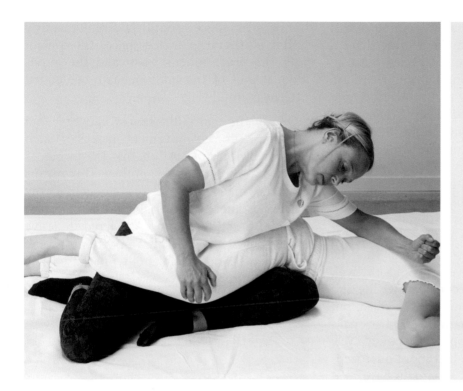

Fig. 2.1
Proprioception and interoception for both the practitioner and the recipient.

Being able to understand one's internal experience and to identify at that level with oneself can be one of the very positive outcomes of having regular Thai massages with an experienced and highly skilled practitioner.

Thai massage focuses on Sên, pathways of movement in the body which are stimulated via the channels (see Chapter 10). This aspect of the work could explain why there is such a strong impact on interoception – the nerves are being woken up. The Thai medicine approach to massage is different to a Western one, which in turn alters outcomes. The practitioner focuses on generating the movement of Wind through the Sên of the recipient's body, which is hugely significant as a physiological aspect of the treatment.

Side note: Channels are spaces between structures or where muscle attaches to bone. They are fascia. Deep to them is Sên.

Sensations felt in the body are caused by thoughts and emotions. We know that all pain is an output of the brain and central nervous system, the two-way highway. If we look at this from the Thai medicine perspective, bodily sensations of pain are communicated from the Sên but originate as an end result of the faster element of Wind (a thought *is* movement; see Chapter 13).

Often, it takes pain, high levels of anxiety, or an intense physical sensation that cannot

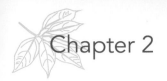

be ignored to alert us that something else is going on. For example, a client might have a vague awareness that she is stressed but carries on regardless, pushing herself. There are small indicators that she continues to ignore as she focuses on her long to-do list. She continues in this way for quite some time until suddenly, with no warning and with nothing particular happening, her back seizes up. She then has to stop and listen to her body. She cannot walk, and is unable to leave the house or "do" anything. It takes a long time for her to heal and return to normal life. During this period of rest, she does some things that she enjoys, which are creative and non-physical. She has lots of time to reconsider her life and think. Many different emotions surface, but after a month she feels changed. Her back pain made her reassess and stop the perpetual cycle that she was in. Had she had more interoceptive awareness earlier on, she might have been able to avoid the pain and make changes to her life without the suffering. Eventually, her body gave her the message "STOP! – you haven't been listening." It took a big, impactful problem to make her notice herself.

Developing interoception, listening deeply to the internal landscape, *is* self-protection and self-care. As practitioners, this is a key component of our businesses, for maintaining the health of our own mind and body, and for facilitating deeper interoceptive listening for the people we work with and support.

Have you ever considered that you get a sense of yourself as you move through your external environment? You know yourself by all that you are not. At times, throughout a treatment, the receiver's body is moved systematically through space, allowing it to passively explore the negative space around it, simultaneously feeling all that it is in that space. The contact with the practitioner's body and the gravitational pull of the floor beneath are added external stimuli (Fig. 2.2).

One of the many differences between Thai massage and self-movement practices such as **Reusi Dat Ton** (RDT) is that the former is given by one person to another. This means that the experience of movement for the receiver is altered and triggers different areas of brain function to those triggered in active movement such as RDT. Importantly, some movements are possible only because they

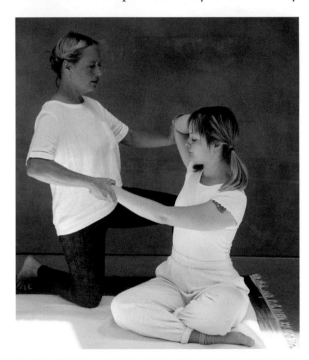

Fig. 2.2
A different experience of movement when it is applied.

are being applied. Alongside this, touch is an enormously effective tool that can provide new cerebral sensations and perceptions of one's own body. Simple touch alone is powerful: an embrace, a pat on the back, even a shake of the hand can break down the walls we create around ourselves and enable self-connection.

Thai massage addresses the body in many ways, including bringing together touch and movement. Stretching, shaking, vibration, range of motion, and skilled touch can awaken self-awareness for the recipient, and an experience of their own body in the present. Working directly on the pathways of movement in the body, known in Thai theory collectively as Sên (nerves, arteries, tendons, ligaments, and so on), gets the Winds moving physically, emotionally, and mentally, and it is common for the recipient to experience a newly awakened and deepened perception of themselves. Long-held and deep compressions, performed with skill and attentiveness, invoke a profound internal awareness for the recipient.

Wind Gate work can stimulate the deepest aspects of the body by working gently on internal structures that developed first in the embryo and are therefore are an "old" part of us, with a lifetime of stored memories.

Through this intense physical focus, the receiver experiences movement without effort or engaging motor control. This can be a vastly different experience, where range of motion increases, or pain levels reduce or disappear completely. Despite the massage being strong, because the layers of the body have been sufficiently addressed it is common for the recipient to start to experience a deep, restful state with many physiological changes occurring.

Touch Perception

Touch is one of the most basic and primal expressions of care, being so innate that we do not need science or research to verify its efficacy. Touch is a natural human communication that is instinctive in all of us, yet it is interesting to gain an understanding of what might be going on under the skin.

The somatosensory system is a vast network of sensory nerve endings located in our skin and fascia, and through which we have the sense of touch. In Thai medicine, nerves are categorized as Sên (pathways of movement in the body; see Chapter 10 for more). We need to keep our bodies moving, balanced, hydrated, and nourished for optimum signaling throughout this system.

Receptors are cells that respond to stimulus and send impulses to sensory nerves. This system, often known as "touch perception," has four main receptors:

- **Mechanoreceptors** send signals about sensations such as pressure, texture, and pain; the palms, feet, fingertips, and most connective tissues are rich in these receptors.

- **Thermoreceptors** communicate information about temperature.

- **Nociceptors** are found in the skin, connective tissue, muscles, organs, bone, and blood vessels, and keep the body safe by detecting pain. **Nociception** is the process by which they send "danger threat" signals to the brain, which then has the task of discerning how real and dangerous the threat is, and what action (if any) to take.

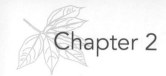

- **Proprioceptors** are located in the tendons, muscles, and joints, and sense changes in muscle tension and length.

When we touch the body and press, rub, or move the skin and underlying tissues, we stimulate these receptors, which then send signals along the neural pathways from the skin to the spinal cord, and then to the control center of the brain. The brain recognizes that something has happened and evaluates what that might be, before sending out its own impulses along the nerves to effect a change. If the initial input (the touch) is pleasant and not seen as a threat, the body will respond to this by relaxing, releasing tension, slowing down breathing, decreasing pain: a parasympathetic nervous response has been triggered. However, if the touch seems to be a threat, the body will respond by doing the exact opposite, triggering a fight or flight response. Touch does not have to be deep to invoke a response throughout the whole body.

A pain response or a danger signal triggered by the nociceptors should not happen in a therapeutic environment. The body does not respond well to a painful touch experience.

"Many currently utilized therapeutic massage techniques unnecessarily inflict patient pain and exacerbate the patient's condition, due to a faulty and erroneous viewpoint regarding biological sensory input and proprioceptors."

Gregory T. Lawton, 2001

Both sadly and incorrectly, Thai massage has long had the reputation of being deep to the point of pain, sending out the wrong kind of signaling to the brain and rest of the body. Thai massage *can* be very deep if that is the level of pressure that feels good to the recipient and the layer being worked on is ready for it. The practitioner must stimulate mechanoreceptors, not nociceptors. However, the effectiveness of "subtleties of touch" is important to acknowledge. Stuck tissue that has no movement in it will need patient touch that slowly creates space and fluidity. If it can be worked this way, it will not resist touch or set up a counterproductive pain response.

"Deep tissue techniques should be applied first with a gentle pressure into the tissue for a depth of one to three centimeters (to stimulate the mechanoreceptors), then to the depth of the periosteum or joint complex."

Gregory T. Lawton, 2009

Side note: If you see your client writhing in pain or trying to get away from your massage work, this is a definite indicator that a fight or flight central nervous system response has been activated and you should back off immediately.

"Proper application of medical massage technique should include the avoidance of technique that stimulates nociceptive responses in the nervous system. This stimulation has a negative effect on the outcome of the treatment and the patient's healing process. From this viewpoint, pain is not gain."

Gregory T. Lawton, 2009

Optimal Level of Pressure – Touch Receptors

We know that the brain, skin, and nervous system all evolved from the first embryonic cells. We cannot separate the body into parts and must understand that when we touch the body, we affect each and every cell and function, because everything is intimately interlinked (Fig. 2.3). As practitioners, we aim to treat our clients with integrity, working with them, not on them. The internal processes that are triggered from the simplicity of touch are worth reflecting on from a wider perspective.

The word "pressure" is most often associated with some kind of force, power, or strength. In fact, the *Concise Oxford English Dictionary* (1988) gives this description: "exertion of continuous force, so exerted upon or against a body by another in contact with it." Yet during Thai massage, we do not want to use force, power, or any type of pressure that harms, hurts, or pushes the body.

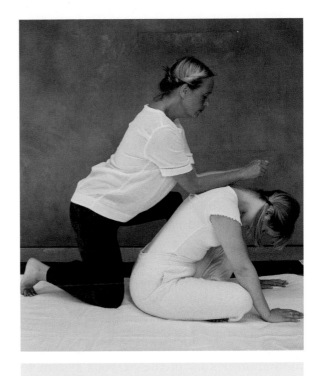

Fig. 2.3
Two forearms creating a **myofascial** stretch between the shoulder blades.

It is by using *aware* and *mindful* touch that the practitioner can execute optimal pressure that affects the whole body therapeutically. This type of touch is one that can reach the Sên, creating communication and movement without causing pain or harm. The Sên are not superficial and so touch has to reach the layer in which they located, with hands that *sink* into the body to reach them effectively (see Chapter 18).

Chapter 2

"Pressure is a physical force, which is used by massage practitioners to achieve therapeutic results. Thus, the therapist converts the kinetic energy of massage strokes into various physiological phenomena on tissue and cellular levels of the body (e.g. changes of **interstitial** pressure), as well as into a chain of electrochemical reactions in the massaged area and the whole organism."

Ross Turchaninov, 2000

Recent research suggests that touch which is pleasant and comfortable is more likely to be effective and therapeutic. Conscious touch and listening hands allow the body to respond with a positive reaction in the tissues, and activates mechanoreceptors in the nervous system to send constant impulses to the brain and back again. It is the communication in the nervous system that ultimately controls the softening of tissue and the pleasurable sensation of Wind releasing or movement created.

Pressure that hits the "sweet spot," finding the exact and perfect level of satisfying touch, results in a more profound response than an overly deep and forced, prolonged, or painful pressure. This pleasurable touch, which is certainly able to be strong or deep, feels good; it might even be described as exquisite pain. This is not really pain that hurts, but it is a definite satisfying sensation and experience of going deep into the tissue to release and affect the Wind element.

Yet if the client is grimacing or tensing up, then the likelihood is that the application of touch is going too deep and is therefore unlikely to be therapeutic. It could be causing the body to feel threatened, which causes stress and is counterproductive. Some may also see this "trying to get away" as a fight or flight response that would involve stress chemicals and tension, not the parasympathetic response of resting and repair.

As practitioners of this healing art, we do not like to learn that clients have had a bad experience of massage, yet we often do hear this about Thai and other modalities. Unfortunately, what we hear is that pressure was too deep or strong. Sometimes, it seems that parts of the treatment were *really* unpleasant, which might make us wonder why a practitioner would think this therapeutic, or if they are using an application of compassionate touch.

There are clients who seem to need to feel discomfort or pain to believe they have had their money's worth, or that it was the deep pressure that made the session effective, an attitude that we as practitioners should challenge. It could be that they follow the outdated philosophy of "no pain no gain," in which case some re-education is perhaps required. Maybe they think they feel good during or immediately after the session, but is this due to pain-relieving **endorphins** being produced and activated, or is it that they feel they have been sufficiently "worked on" for a change to have been facilitated? Perhaps they have become disconnected from sensing the subtleties in their body, or even display a level of numbness. They may not yet be aware that refined approaches such as heart–mind work could lead to a parasympathetic nervous system response whereby the body begins to rest and repair. As the Winds in the body are calmed and reactivated, the body wakes up to sensation.

Some clients are not in touch with their own body and because of this they may feel numb. This is why working through the layers is beneficial. Start superficial and go deeper as the body allows it, instead of pressing in to try to stimulate a sensation. The deep work can encourage a profound self-awareness, but it is not always possible to work deeply in initial sessions if the practitioner is truly listening.

Consider the analogy of a pebble in a pond. If we throw the pebble in such a way that it skims the surface of the water, we can see ripples spreading outwards for quite some distance. To skim the pebble in this way requires some skill or practice, but creates far-reaching movement. If we took the same pebble and threw it hard into the water, it creates a temporarily satisfying noise, but then disappears quickly without leaving a lasting impression on the surrounding water. Our fluid bodies might also respond to being touched in a skillful yet gentle way, and they respond best to a type of touch that acknowledges the many layers deeper within, by sinking into them, appreciating and spending time on each layer. The most powerful and healing approach is to do less with invitation and more with force.

We need to keep our intention clear. What are we trying to achieve? Is a big, deep, intense approach to the body going to be the one that creates the most change or potential for healing? Or can we actually work with an intelligent touch, listening moment by moment to what we feel is going to be most helpful for the individual client, within the functional passive limitations of their body in the present moment? It may be that they feel they want intense pressure from the outset, but when they receive touch to the skin before addressing the deeper layers one by one, it meets the frequency of their body, which will be experienced as a deeper, more profound, treatment.

In giving Thai massage this way, we can make use of the big, bold, deep techniques, such as compressions and stretches, because sometimes they are what is needed. When the range of pressure required favors the deeper end of the spectrum, it can be facilitated by correct body mechanics, not by "pushing" the body into pain. But equally, knowing when to back off and be happy to encourage the body slowly and gently to release and let go in its own time, with no force, means that we are really connected with the client. Working in this way, we are taking the lead from their body in the present moment, rather than following their initial instruction or our own ego.

There may be times when the tension that clients feel in their body is so acute that it seems as if the only way to release it is with prolonged forced pressure or an intensified stretch. This may seem good in the moment, but in the long run it does not encourage the body to heal itself. When clients are already in pain, they do not need more pain to make them better – there is no logic to this! The tissues need to

be touched with intelligence and curiosity, exploring the area to coax movement into it. There is a big difference between forced hard pressure and a compression that leans into the area, slowly sinking in without force.

Pressure that is given through the use of gravity, movement, and sensitive touch does heal. Using the weight of the body in this way, finding a slow, unhurried, steady pace, is what works best. Fascia needs time and responds to intelligent pressure that eases in and out.

Side note: A psychic healer described the strong impact that light touch has on the body, and his words are always in my mind when I am touching someone who is frail, numb to sensation, or disconnected from this idea of thought impacting emotion impacting outcome.

"Very light pressure causes compression on an energetic and subtle level. This puts form with form or like with like, getting atoms and molecules to register a liquid within a liquid state."

Michael Jenkins, personal communication, 2017

This simple viewpoint and gentle touch intention have had huge effects in my clinic. When someone is in pain or asks for extremely deep pressure, I often find that a "less is more" approach is more powerful and therapeutic in the long run.

PART 2

The Body

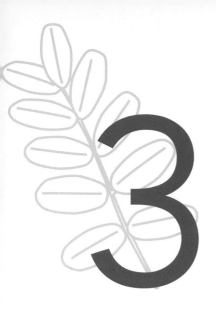

3

The Body, Nature, and Thai Anatomy

Before we delve into some Thai element theory, it is important to explain the context a little first.

Thai anatomy looks at the body through a very different lens to a Western one. It has many component parts, some of which I have included below. Bear in mind that this is not an exhaustive list by any stretch of the imagination.

Thai anatomy is comprised of the layers of the physical body, the three aspects, **Kwan**, five elements, essence, Sên theory, **release points**, heart–mind, **Wind Gate**, and food and waste products. These are described in further chapters in more detail.

Element theory is a vast subject, one that you could literally study for years. It is a deeply interesting, insightful, and inspiring way to see the body and understand it in a very different way. In this book I am going to convey some very basic knowledge of the Thai element system.

The elements come primarily from Buddha's teachings, ancient medical texts, and meditations. Practitioners of medicine would meditate on the elements to gain deep understanding and then would record their insights and pass on knowledge.

Religion and medicine merged together in Asia, and more specifically in Thailand. Thai medicine is fundamentally Buddhist medicine, but of course not all Buddhist medicine is from Thailand. The teachings of the Buddha, called **Buddha Dhamma**, are practiced widely throughout Asia. In each country, the culture, flora and fauna, and different spiritual practices had a big influence on the development of medicine there. We can see from this how different systems developed and evolved, but how, at a glance, they seem similar.

Throughout this book I will touch briefly on element theory and other components of Thai anatomy, and you will find further resources at the back of the book for more in-depth study.

The Elements in Thai Medicine

The five elements are Earth, Water, Fire, Wind, and Space. Consciousness is sometimes grouped together with Space and at other times is classed as a sixth element.

When I first learned that there was element theory in Thai medicine, I was delighted. I was finally able to uncover the theory that I had been seeking to give depth to my bodywork practice.

Chapter 3

Many years ago, when studying nutrition, I learned about elements through the Chinese five-element system; it always made so much sense to me to perceive the body (and to know how to treat it) from this perspective.

Metal and Wood are components of the Chinese system but are not part of Thai medicine. There are, of course, other variants that make Thai theory different to any other system, but one thing is certain: the bodywork techniques produce astounding results when approached through this lens and not mixed up with others.

The Buddha taught about elements in a simple way, knowing the obvious connections and similarities between the body and the natural world. The elements are the same, whether we look at the internal landscape or the external one. They have the same experience, function, and quality.

Earth and Water make up the anatomy of the body.

Fire and Wind make up the physiology of the body.

Experience

The experience of Earth is solidity. This makes it very tangible and dense, so that things cannot pass through it.

The experience of Water is wateriness, liquidity. Water makes things malleable and it binds.

The experience of Fire is heat, and it transforms things and ripens them.

The experience of Wind is movement, vibration, and growth.

Function

Earth provides resistance and support. We can put things on it; it has the function of giving support, so we can step on the ground and not fall through it. We can put a cup on the table and it will be supported by the table.

Water provides cohesion and fluidity. It enables things to be supple and flexible. When you add water to things, it binds them together and makes them more malleable. For example: if water is added to flour, it sticks together and becomes pliable.

Fire transforms things. The fruit on the tree ripens through heat, transforming from being unripe to being ripe, and eventually decaying. Food changes its molecular structure when heated, and can burn if there is too much heat.

Wind moves; the movement has a vibration. A seed grows up from the ground, a fetus develops in utero, and an idea comes to fruition, due to Wind. Even the smallest movement that one might see under a microscope, the smallest of vibrations, is Wind element.

Quality

Earth is stable and heavy. It is dense and immobile.

Water is moist, fluid, soft, and able to move (although it does not move unless Wind moves it). Water has the potential to be manipulated.

Fire is bright, reactive, and sharp. If you were to touch fire, the sensation of the heat would be sharp.

Wind is light, mobile, and dry. Wind is the only element that moves any of the other elements. Wind is not heavy; it is the lightest of elements.

Temperature

Each element has a temperature association, which becomes very important when working with medicine and choosing bodywork tools. Any hot condition would be treated with cooling herbs and techniques, whereas a cold condition would need warmth and heat to create balance and good health.

Earth is mild, neither hot or cold.

Water is ice-cold.

Fire is hot.

Wind is cool (and as it moves, you could think of it like a breeze).

There is no temperature associated with Space element.

Sense Connected to Element

Earth

- Sense organ: the nose – smell.

- Earth can be felt, heard, seen, tasted and smelled.

Water

- Sense organ: the mouth – taste.

- Water can be felt, heard, seen, and tasted.

Fire

- Sense organ: eyes – sight.

- Fire can be heard, felt, and seen, but not tasted or smelled.

Wind

- Sense organ: skin – touch.

- Wind can be heard and felt, but cannot been seen, touched, or smelled.

How Are the Elements Represented in Us?

The physical body has both Earth and Water characteristics. These are the most physical and tangible aspects of our anatomy.

Emotions are represented by Water and Fire elements.

Fire and Wind are the elements attributed to our thoughts and the mental aspect.

Space is the element attributed to consciousness, the spirit, and the soul.

Anatomy

Earth and Water make the physical body: they are our gross anatomy.

Chapter 3

There are twenty Earth body parts, such as the skin, muscles, bones, and organs (listed below). Water has twelve body parts, such as bile, tears, **synovial fluid**, and blood, which give the experience of being in a fluid state. Combined, they make up thirty-two parts of the gross, physical body.

These two elements have a close relationship with each other and also share similar characteristics, in that they are the slowest and heaviest of the elements (Earth being the heaviest). They represent the body in its most physical form.

Function/Physiology

Fire and Wind are the movements of the body from gross to subtle, as well as the impetus for things to happen, the breath you take, the beat of the heart, the drive you have, the thousands of thoughts running through your mind, your metabolic processes, the transformation of food into energy. They are our physiology, the energetic functioning of the body, much like a house has energy running through it in the form of heat and electricity. You cannot touch these elements but they act on Earth and Water.

The Fifth Element

Space is expansive yet subtle. The subtlety of it often leads to it not being given much thought, for how often do we notice the negative Space around us? Despite this, Space is always present as a field for all other elements to exist in; it is the element of becoming, from which all other elements take life and form. It is the negative Space around us, the spaciousness in our body when we feel, move, and live healthily, the Space between cells, the open Spaces in the body such as the nostrils and mouth, and the Space we try to create in our minds with meditation. The experience of Space is that it is unobstructed.

Space is fast-moving (quantum physics talks about there being Space between matter and about it having unlimited potential). This is the lightest of all elements; it is not tangible and has no resistance.

Earth – Din

There are twenty body parts associated with Earth (**Din**). These represent the structure of the body parts, not the function of them. When we are talking about Earth body parts, we are describing the muscles themselves, not their function while they contract or decelerate. We are talking about the lungs, not their function or movement as a breath is taken. We are looking at the physical structure of tendons and ligaments themselves, not their purpose as pathways of movement. These are the body parts that provide support and solidity. All things solid in the body are Earth element, including any organs and structures not listed here. You can see on the list opposite that the twenty Earth components are ordered from superficial to deep, and from the head to the feet (see also Fig. 3.1).

The twenty Earth component parts

1. Hair on head

2. Hair on body

3. Nails

4. Teeth

5. Skin

6. Muscles

7. Sên (tendons, ligaments, nerves, blood vessels)

8. Bone

9. Marrow

10. Kidneys

11. Heart

12. Liver

13. Fascia (in some texts this refers to the **pleura**)

14. Spleen

15. Lungs

16. Large intestine

17. Small intestine

18. Stomach and new food

19. Feces

20. Brain and central nervous system.

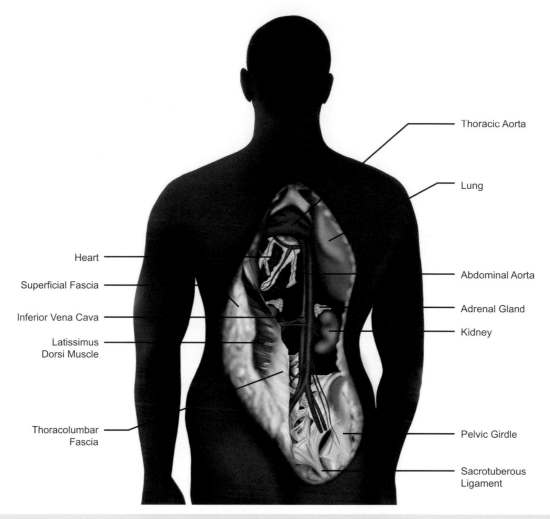

Fig. 3.1
Posterior view of Earth element body parts.

Water – Nam

As the name suggests, Water element (**Nam**) is the anatomy of the body related to its fluids and the experience of being liquid. Anything that has a fluid nature is Water element: the sweat on our skin, the tears we cry, the blood in our veins, the saliva we swallow, the synovial fluid of our joints. It is also the *potential* for malleability and flexibility in the tissues and structures. The function of Water is that it is cohesive and fluid. If you imagine two drops of water, they will bind to each other because this element has a sticky nature.

The twelve Water component parts

1. Bile

2. Mucus in the respiratory tract

3. Pus and lymph

4. Blood

5. Sweat

6. Fat (the harder fats such as superficial fascia)

7. Tears

8. Oil (such as the grease on skin and inside the body)

9. Saliva

10. Mucus in the nose/throat

11. Synovial fluid

12. Urine.

Fire – Fai

Heat transforms things: from not ripe to ripe, from raw to cooked. The fruit on a tree ripens and then decays because of the heat of the sun. The heat of Fire (**Fai**) breaks down food so that the body can use it.

The four Fire component parts

1. Fire that causes aging and decay; it is responsible for the breakdown of toxins and blood in the liver, as well as the aging process.

2. Fire that provides warmth; it is our body temperature and causes us to need to cool down, bathe ourselves, and feel hunger and thirst.

3. Fire of digestion that is responsible for the breakdown of food and any other digestive process in the body. We can use bile as an example (although it is listed as a Water component part): it is the heat of Fire and its transformative function that cause the breakdown of food.

4. Fire that causes emotion and fever.

Wind – Lom

Wind (**Lom**) is the movement of *all* things in the body. It is a light and subtle element. Anything that moves, from gentle and subtle to the biggest and most dramatic of movements, is Wind element expressing itself.

The six wind component parts

1. Ascending Wind that moves from the feet to the head (as in burping, vomiting, words). (Some ancient texts talk about the ascending Wind which moves specifically from the navel to the top of the head, and is a primary Wind for balance and prevention of disease.)

2. Wind that moves from the top of the head to the feet (as in menstruation, childbirth, defecation, urination). (The ancient texts also refer to the descending Wind which moves specifically from the navel to the feet, and is a primary one for balance and disease prevention.)

3. Wind that is within the digestive tract. This is the Wind that we swallow when we eat and that pushes food from mouth to anus.

4. Wind within the abdomen but outside the digestive tract; all Wind that moves the organs in the torso.

5. Wind that circulates to all parts of the body, including the extremities, such as nervous impulses and blood through blood vessels.

6. Wind that is inhaled and exhaled.

Side note: The ancient texts that categorize the ascending and descending Winds together, and as starting at the navel, speak of the interaction between them being a great influence on the health and temperature of blood, which is a real indicator of vitality in Thai medicine.

Space

Space element, in relation to the body, is all those areas of us that have a connection between the internal and the external.

The Space component parts

There are ten Space component parts in women and nine in men:

1. Eyes (two)

2. Ears (two)

3. Nostrils (two)

4. Mouth

5. Anus

6. Urethra

7. Vagina.

Experience, Function, and Quality

- Experience: unobstructedness.

- Function: non-resistance and field of activity for other elements.

- Qualities: expansive, subtle.

Elements in Relation to Bodywork

The structure of the diaphragm is Earth element. Taking a deep breath creates movement (Wind) in the respiratory tract; the movement of the respiratory organs is Wind, although the organs themselves are Earth element, for they are a container and have a solid aspect to them. The heat of the breath indicates Fire, and the malleability of the lungs indicates that Water element is present.

A muscle's structure is Earth element. The fluid surrounding the muscle tissue is Water element, but the movement of it when being stretched is Wind element, and warmth in the muscle is Fire element. A deep compression or squeezing of the muscle will encourage an exchange of fluid (Water element) in the tissue, but the movement of the fluid is Wind element. The heat that is generated through touch is Fire element, while the movement of the blood through Sên to the skin is Wind element.

In Thai bodywork, understanding the elements is key. Let's take a look at them in turn in more detail.

Earth

Earth element is the slowest and densest part of us, such as bone, organs, and skin. Similar to the Earth's core, there is a dense solidity to this element in the body. If the practitioner feels hard, bound-up areas of muscle tissue, Earth element is agitated. When the body develops bony protrusions or calcifications such as a bunion, this is amplified Earth element. A tumor is deranged Earth element.

Water

Water is a fluid and sticky substance, and is cohesive. A chest full of mucus indicates amplified Water, whereas constipation primarily indicates depleted Water. (It can also indicate depleted Wind element, as the feces are slow to move.)

Fire

Fire is both heat and lack of heat. It has many attributes associated with it, such as motivation, power, and anger. It will generate or initiate movement, whether on a physical or an emotional level. In the physical body, this element is one of transformation and transmutation. It is the element related to hormones: that is, aging, decay, and maturation. It is also commonly seen as the element for passion and strong feelings, but conversely is seen in its depleted state as emotional coldness or lack of excitement – a lack of Fire.

Wind

Wind is not to be confused with the **Ayurvedic** element of Air. Air is still, while Wind moves and has a mobile nature. Wind is responsible for all the body's major physiological movements. Here are some functional examples of how this element represents kinetic energy in the body.

Wind is the circulation of blood and body fluids. Wind stimulates excretion of all digestive enzymes. It is all metabolic processes and the **peristaltic** movement of the intestines. It is neurotransmitters, the carrier of your voice, the experience of touch as it is communicated along the neural pathways (Sên) to the brain. It is the monkey-mind, thoughts so fast and subtle they often go unnoticed.

Wind is the element in us that is most easily thrown out of balance, but also, being the lightest element of human physiology, the easiest to bring back to balance. If the Wind fluctuates in an irregular way, it can cause a disturbance such as fainting.

If we think about the universe as a mirror, we can see that Wind element relates to movement in the atmosphere: both a subtle breeze and a howling gale have a noticeable impact. Anxiety can tip someone over the edge with cascading effects on sleep patterns, digestion, emotional balance. Wind possesses the ability to be unpredictable and create chaos, yet has vast potential to quickly become balanced as it is so light.

A stiff, immobile body has impeded Wind on a gross (physical) level. An anxious thought is agitated Wind on a subtle (non-physical) level. There are gross and subtle movements of Wind in the body: imagine the movement of a hormone (subtle) and acknowledge this movement, then compare it to the movement of your body as you dance. In this comparison we can observe that both are movements, but on a macro/micro level.

Side note: The monkey-mind is one that swings around, restless, agitated, and unsettled. It is a great example of how Wind causes mental havoc.

Space

There is a reason why humans need to go into the outdoors. We need to feel the Space around us, to feel free of the heavy confines of walls, bricks, and mortar. It is natural to search for a sense of Space and freedom not found in a man-made, built-up environment. More people also seek Space in their minds, and meditation and mindfulness are becoming increasingly popular due to the necessity for unobstructedness, from which one can gain clarity and peace.

Similarly, there needs to be a feeling of spaciousness inside our bodies. This is so that every organ, all the fasciae, every ligament, tendon, muscle, and all other internal structures can function freely. If tissues get stuck in the body without sufficient differential movement, when there is constriction and adhesions, we start to see problems in function occurring or pain developing. For example, the lungs are perched on top of the diaphragm, with fascia separating them from each other. Ideally, each breath taken expands and contracts the lungs, which massage the diaphragm and liver, but if there has been inflammation and the fascia is restricted and stuck around the lungs, or between the diaphragm and lungs, there could be limited slide and glide so that sufficient differential movement is impossible.

There is potential in Space as atoms and molecules are further apart and faster-moving. When we have more Space in our tissues, when we have been given Space to relax or let go, we feel better. When the mind is full or cluttered, it has a direct impact on the rest of the body. As Space is created in the tissues, Wind can move through the channels, blood can flow, and the body can more easily absorb nutrients and experience greater freedom.

Thai massage practitioners create a sense of Space in the body through various techniques that relax and release bound-up tension or tightness in the muscles and fascia. As these tissues alter their structure and become more malleable, there is a knock-on effect on the subsequent layers, creating more Space for unimpeded function. This results in a substantial feeling of Space and unobstructedness where there was heaviness and rigidity. Traction creates Space between two bony structures.

Elements Concentrated

- *Earth* – pelvis; a heavy and dense structure, a mid point between the upper and lower body.

- *Water* – belly; a fluid, malleable and soft area.

- *Fire* – liver and gallbladder; notorious for the heat of bile, which helps break things down and transform them.

- *Wind* – heart and lungs; think of their constant movement, the in and out breath, the pulsation of the heart.

- *Space* – the mind.

Elements Coming into Existence

We need to look at the elements as they come into existence because it helps us to understand the patterns of how they can manifest in the body, how they condense and solidify, and can be dispersed. This is particularly helpful during bodywork, as we can make choices more easily.

This is the understanding of the creation of matter, which comes first from Consciousness and then Space.

There are subtle Winds of Consciousness, which, as they grow stronger, gather momentum (and create a desire or intent). This movement picks up impetus, which then causes friction. This friction creates heat, and as it meets cold it causes condensation. (Heat is warm, Wind is cool, so the heat outside and the cool inside create condensation.) This goes on to produce dampness, which becomes stagnant through lack of movement and eventually crystallizes, becoming solid, which is Earth element.

This pattern is the same in the disease process. Habitual tendencies, **karma**, the movement of thoughts in the mind become more substantial and then eventually develop into an emotion which affects the physical structures and function of the body (that is, the body is the end result of thought and feeling).

The anxious thought that becomes loose stools; the excitement of falling in love that becomes butterflies in the stomach; bile that rises up as we become angry or bitter: if they continue, all of these thoughts become physical and affect the more physical aspects of us (Water and Earth).

To understand disease through the Thai system, we look at Water, Fire, and Wind. Wind is the lightest and easiest element to balance, whereas Earth is the structure of the body, less to do with disease and more to do with digestion and organ health.

The Universe and the Body Mirrored

Going into the **cadaver** lab for the first time, I *really* saw that there is a whole world going

on inside us. I saw the layers of the body, the patterns, textures, and their depths like the layers of the earth, the fluids like the rivers, the shapes of human form just like the undulating hills.

Inside the body there are spaces, crevices, and caverns, solid and dense structures, continuations from superficial to deep that are so far-reaching that you can see how connected everything is, inside and out. There are depths where you can get lost so easily that landmarks are needed during the explorations into human form in a lab. There is organization and beauty so unexpected in the body, yet our lives often go by without us ever really taking time to reflect on this. Instead, we may find ourselves searching our external environment, finding beauty there, easily forgetting that everything is truly reflected inside us. All the familiar sights of the world are reflections of our own form if we choose to see it that way.

The layers of the body cannot truly be separated from each other because nothing is really separate. The elements, both of the body and of the natural world, are not isolated. They exist and are at play all the time, waxing and waning, varying in their vibrancy or quality, which is what distinguishes them from each other. For example, the water in a river may be cold (Water is a cold element), yet it has the potential to warm up (so it must have some Fire in it). The river may be fast-flowing or almost still; either way, if there is any movement at all, or potential for movement, Wind is displaying itself. The solid banks of the river contain the water. Solidity is the experience of Earth element. Everything, be it in the natural world or the body, has the experience, function, and quality of all the elements – Earth, Water, Fire, Wind, and Space; they just display themselves in differing states.

Each element can be observed in nature with the same qualities, function, and experience it presents in the body. If you study the landscape around you and compare it to your internal landscape, you will see that the water in the stream has the same qualities as the tears that fall down your face, fluid in nature. The movement of Wind that creates ripples on the surface of the water has the same quality of movement as the Wind that moves the blood through your body. The element that heats the water in the stream, making it possible to dip your toes in, is Fire and it is this element that warms the blood in your veins. The solid container that holds the water in the river bank is Earth, like the muscle and bone that provide solidity for your body. The stream is restrained from bursting its banks by the solidity of earth, just as the blood in the vessels of the body is contained by fascia, one of the twenty body parts of Earth element.

Side note: Notice the trees around you, how they are solid and dense, how they can withstand the strongest of winds. Notice how a wind that is unrelenting and fierce can eventually break the tree and it falls, in the same way that Wind can cause pain and create havoc with posture or function.

Observe how heavy rain causes the earth to swell and lose its solidity as it soaks up water, in the same way that our bodies can swell with conditions like **edema**. Both the muddy earth and the body in these states can have a similar consistency.

The sun's heat can scorch the earth, start fires, and melt snow. It can accelerate aging of the skin, make tempers rise, and warm the blood that runs through our bodies. Fire can create havoc in the body, as it can on our planet. It can cause fevers or chills and hormonal imbalances that have a knock-on effect, just as it impacts the global eco-system.

Wind can produce chaos, taking down trees and houses in its path. It can literally whip people off their feet. This element can play havoc with an already anxious mind, make someone so restless that they cannot settle, and send knife-like pains through the body. Without it, clothes on the line do not dry and bodies stiffen and lose mobility.

Wind in the body is the element most strongly associated with pain. There are winds that move the subtle and gross around the body (called the heart wind), winds that cause pain (knife-like wind), and the winds of the central channel in the spinal column, vena cava and aorta. They are the trunks of the nerve and heart trees, gross Sên that support all life-giving movement in the body.

Essence

While, in traditional theory, the essence of the body is described as a golden liquid permeating the organs, especially the heart, I have not seen this gold fluid myself during a dissection. I once asked my teacher, Gil, about it, as he has dissected hundreds of bodies, some of them unfixed (an unfixed cadaver has not been embalmed), and he also was not aware of any such golden liquid. However, perhaps this description is symbolic, a color and consistency used to define its vitality, potential, and health.

Essence in a healthy body can be seen with someone who glows, radiates good health, and has vital energy. You could perceive this in young children, who are at a watery element time of life and are in the process of fully becoming.

Essence can be depleted by unhealthy daily habits that affect the immune system, but also by menstruation and ejaculation.

Essence can be nourished by foods that are mostly sweet and replenishing.

Later in this book (Chapter 15), you will find a recipe for golden milk, which is wonderfully warming and nourishes essence. Other foods that help replenish essence are dates, honey, maple syrup, almonds, and Brazil nuts. Women also benefit from tonifying herbs, keeping warm (belly binding to keep the kidneys and other internal organs warm), and resting during **menarche** (see Chapter 24).

Poor daily habits will affect essence and deplete the natural vitality of the body. Late nights and not enough sleep, over-consumption of stimulants, and stress will directly affect the endocrine and immune systems,

which will have the adverse effect of depleting essence.

Blood

In traditional Thai medicine, blood is viewed as indicative of health, as it carries vital nutrients around the whole body. Its movement along pathways and throughout the body epitomizes it as the essence of life. Its color and consistency can also be used diagnostically in practices such as **cupping**.

Side note: Black blood that is drawn to the surface during cupping is seen as stagnant, while deep red indicates heat pathogen, and pale blood is considered to be depleted.

Blood is an unusual substance, as it has three element components: it has the heat of Fire element, the movement of Wind element, and the liquidity of Water element.

If the blood is not circulating in a healthy way, it will signify Wind element not being balanced. If the blood is stagnant, fatty, or toxic, then its Water element component is out of balance. The temperature of the blood indicates the health of Fire element.

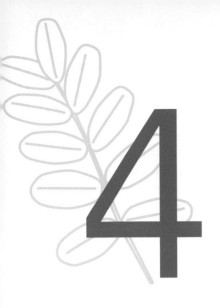

4 Bodywork for the Element Types

There are many specific techniques and considerations that influence treatment choices and which depend on **core element constitution** (CEC; see Chapter 5) and current imbalances. While they are loose guidelines, and only one aspect of how to apply the bodywork, they should influence how you work to maximize healing potential.

When even a very basic understanding of Thai element theory is bought into a Thai bodywork session, the efficacy can be transformational, as it addresses the needs of an individual and their current imbalances.

There are techniques that work for some element body types and not others. Each type will have a preferred depth of pressure or how they like to receive bodywork. What works for one will not for another: one man's medicine is another's poison. All the techniques need to be taught in a classroom with a teacher present. Some techniques involve tools and props, and these should be covered only once a deeper level of study has been achieved.

There are various states of imbalance that play out in the body. A practitioner can choose to balance, nourish, support, diminish, strengthen, and build elements through bodywork and will learn when to use particular

techniques to do this most effectively. The nourishing and supportive techniques will help to build and strengthen someone who is weak, while the balancing and weakening ones will assist those who are agitated and over-stimulated.

Element theory as a whole is a vast subject and one that takes years of study to get to grips with. There are many aspects, including CEC, elemental causes of imbalance, effects of elements on the physical and emotional body, the natural states of imbalance, and many more.

In all bodywork sessions, Earth element is being treated and so there are no specific protocols or therapies to address it or single it out. However, Earth element is slow and heavy (much like Water) and techniques that calm Water element will benefit Earth. We can also pay additional attention to the feet, as they are the body part that spends most time in close contact with (or on) the ground.

Water Element

Watery tissue feels soft, cold, and spongy, and will bruise easily. Care must be taken not to apply strong pressure with focused and sharp tools, such as the thumbs or elbows, when

Chapter 4

working the channels. Broader pressure is often more comfortable.

If the practitioner needs to work Sên to stimulate the pathways and get Wind moving through them, then ironing technique with a warming balm to glide up and/or down the channels is best. Direction is a factor for consideration and this depends on where the Winds need to be moved (towards the core if depleted, away from the core if bursting with energy, and so on). Generally, when working with a Watery CEC, the direction is towards the core, as this will help move fluids and Wind to that area and assist the body in processing the work. As Water is a slow element and stagnation is common, there is often a need to assist the body to process the work by using manual therapy techniques.

As this is a cold element, Watery people benefit from having heating compresses, oils, and balms applied to their body. As it is also a slow-moving element, it is nourishing and supportive to work at a faster pace, generating fire and energy. The intention is to encourage the fluids in the body to start moving, which will have the effect of clearing stagnation.

Side note: When working at a faster pace, it is still important to hit the **bite** and find the **end-feel** each time a technique is applied. When I observe practitioners working, they often miss the "sweet spot" because they are bouncing out too quickly in their haste to work faster.

Twisting, squeezing, pressing, and stretching are also beneficial for Water element. Gentle channel work can be helpful but care must be taken due to the Watery and easily bruised tissue. There is often a sponge-like texture to Watery bodies, which makes it less easy to adjust deep pressure to the right bite or limit. You will find that your hands sink into the tissue, meeting little resistance, and this can initially be challenging for inexperienced hands.

Cupping, using fire or silicone cups, is often very helpful for dispersing stagnation and toxins, and is balancing for this element.

Fire Element

Fiery people like you to get in there quickly, using fairly or really strong pressure from the outset. I have observed practitioners who think this means that the layers need not be addressed, which is not the case. The layers should always be cared for. My advice is to care for the skin, warming it as usual before going in with deeper second-layer techniques such as deep compressions and beating.

Fire is a reactive element and you will find that this makes bodywork take effect quickly, so there is less time needed for treatment and for bodies to adjust and heal.

In general, avoid using oil. I have noticed that oil does not absorb very well into Fiery skin, which tends to be naturally oilier. Also think of how oil feeds a fire. There is the odd occasion when oil is needed (such as for scraping) and in this instance coconut would be preferable: while still warm, it is the coolest of the medicinally based oils.

The tempo and pace for Fiery people dictate working in a calm but confident way without being too slow. You will find that techniques applied too slowly will easily irritate the Fiery person. Fiery people will often not want a really long treatment session, opting more frequently for regular but shorter sessions. This is because they have a tendency to be always on the go.

Compresses should be used cool and be based on cooling herbs. Strong pressure, strong point work, and deep stretches that are held for longer are beneficial for this element. Use techniques such as scraping and beating to disperse and draw out Fire, and if working directionally to calm or disperse the Fires, work away from the navel to the extremities.

If Fire is presenting itself in a depleted state, work towards the core, using heating oils and hot herbal compresses. Fire in a depleted state could show up as a lack of warmth in the body, or lack of drive.

Wind Element

This is the lightest and fastest of the elements that make up the physiology of the body. It is both the easiest to be thrown out of balance and the easiest to be brought back to balance.

Windy people tend to be sensitive to touch *and* to how they are treated. Work in an aware and balanced way without moving around too much. By this I mean avoid working in a chaotic way, moving from one technique to another or changing limb too often. As Wind is a fast element, it is best to work slowly to calm things down. Windy people are highly sensitive and will feel it if you are not confident, which will unsettle their Winds. Remember that there is a fine line between slow work and work that feels unsure. Address both sides with sequence work, as this is a reassuring pattern that ensures symmetry and will calm agitation to the Winds.

Wind is a dry element and benefits from oils being used. (Oil is Water element and has a heaviness to it which is very beneficial and calming for Wind when it is excited.) Raw cold-pressed sesame is best, as it is warming; second to this, safflower is also helpful (it is just less warming, but is still warm). Slightly wet, hot compresses will nourish this element, but take care that you do not make the compresses so wet that they leave damp patches on the body, which will quickly cool and disrupt the Wind, doing the opposite of what the client needs. Balms and liniments that heat and warm are especially therapeutic for Windy people. Wind Gate work is beneficial, as it resets and calms the whole body, and is also sensitive work to which Windy people are receptive.

If Wind is presenting itself in a weakened state, continue to address both sides of the body to bring balance, but use range of motion and oil work with a more energetic angle.

Space

The element of Space cannot be "treated" with bodywork as such, but bodywork does influence the spaciousness of the mind and can create more spaces between structures in the physical body. When people stop rushing around, are encouraged into a restful state, and are touched with the intention of healing, there is a space for things to unfold.

It is predominantly Buddhism which is the mental health root of Thai medicine and can encourage an uncluttered mind. When we have space in our heads, it creates a connection to the self and others which is calm, healthy, and balanced. For this reason, I include a meditation and a mantra here.

Side note: A **Theravada** Buddhist practice, where focus is brought to the breath as it enters and leaves the body at the nostrils, is a simple meditation to create inner space and quieten the mind. The eyes are usually and traditionally kept open in meditation so that there can be a visual, external focal point.

Side note: Repeating the mantra "Buddho, Buddho, Buddho" is very calming and this can be given to someone as a self-care practice. It is particularly helpful for an anxious state of mind. "Buddho" translates as "awakened."

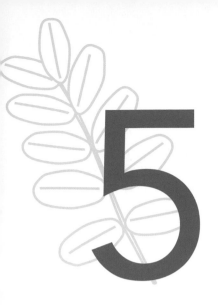

5 Core Element Constitution

From birth, we each have a predominant core constitutional element, which could be described as our own unique natural signature. In other modalities, such as homeopathy, they are called Miasms or genetic traits. Core element constitution (CEC) can reflect our physical appearance and personality traits, mirror the way we react to the environment and other people, and indicate our disease tendencies. In Thai medicine, there is mostly one element that is more prominent than the others. It is how you can look at someone and just *know* they are Fiery; their temper, passion, drive, or coloring may be a loose indicator.

Side note: Core element constitution can be influenced by many factors, such as the time and place of birth, planetary alignment, and parents' genetic traits.

When studied in depth and reflected on, characteristics become easier to recognize in yourself and those around you. This is an intriguing aspect of Thai medicine and people often become heavily fixated on it – more so than any other part of Thai anatomy. Keep in mind that CEC is never a problem; it is just who you are. It does not indicate an imbalance, yet it does help to ascertain how far out of balance someone has become. Understanding someone's CEC can also indicate conditions to which they may be more predisposed. It is also a point of reference for understanding natural inclinations, personality type, and preferences.

Side note: Through bodywork, a change in daily habits, and herbs, we can address imbalances, but we are never trying to change someone's CEC.

When someone's CEC seems less obvious, it is possible that there is a secondary element running alongside the primary one (or even three elements, although this is less common). For example, I always considered myself to be CEC Fire because I am very driven and passionate. I get an idea in my head and see it through to the end, which is a Fiery trait. However, a colleague pointed out that I am actually CEC Wind/Fire, as I am principally a creative person who has lots of ideas – more ideas, in fact, than those that I carry through to the end. It is a typical Windy trait to have lots of ideas, sometimes so many that they can make someone seem very flighty and unfocused. It is the Fire element in me that gets things done. It is not such a Fiery trait to always be working on new ideas and shifting gears.

Side note: Look around you at the world. Notice people, their shapes and sizes, their outlook, temperament, skin, eye and hair color. Observe how they move, speak, and express themselves. All of these and more give clues as to their CEC.

The constitutional element sets around the age of five or six years and then never changes, unless a massive life-changing trauma is experienced at this very early stage. Understanding someone's core element helps the practitioner see how far out of balance that person is when they have a problem. It is the imbalance that is treated with bodywork, not the CEC, because the latter is just "what is" and is not a problem in itself.

Earth – Din

It is pretty rare to have an Earth CEC on its own, but if you do encounter someone with Earth as their core element you will absolutely know them when you see them. They have really big, heavy bones and large, square frames, and they turn heads, not only because of their vast frames but because they tend to be incredibly beautiful and noticeable, although not always in a stereotypical way. They may have big, wide heads, big mouths or teeth, or lots of hair, but they are always somehow striking. Earth types will look like a walking mountain: Lurch from the Addams family, Michelle Obama, and the author and life coach Tony Robbins spring to mind.

Earth types move slowly and have very deep, booming, resonant voices. They are "salt of the earth" people and very grounded. They will be extremely loyal, yet lacking in flexibility. They are slow, in both how they move and how quickly they learn, take on new ideas, or change their point of view; in fact, it is hard to get them to change, as they can be very stubborn. They are generally balanced and compassionate.

Water – Nam

Watery people tend to hold on to water, so lean towards carrying more weight or being fleshier. They have soft, hydrated, healthy, and child-like skin and big, soft eyes, and are often seen as being very beautiful for these reasons. Most often, they will have thick eyelashes and hair, and more hair on their bodies. They tend to suffer more with mucus-related illnesses or are slow to get rid of a cold; they also feel the cold easily and this is a cold element. Water is also a sweet element and Watery people are sweet-natured. Kindness, compassion, and intuition are typical of a Water element person, yet they will lean towards emotions such as worry, nostalgia, depression, and sadness. Watery people bruise easily; their tissue layer is sensitive and spongier. This is a dense and slow element (albeit a little lighter and faster than Earth), and this is reflected in how Watery people take longer to grasp a concept or new idea, or heal slowly. They may have to work a bit harder to learn, but when they do they retain knowledge very well. Watery types, despite being malleable and easy-going, can also get stuck on an idea. They are the glue that holds the family together or brings groups of people together.

Fire – Fai

Someone with Fire as their CEC will have an average physique and will easily build and maintain good musculature. The sense organ of fire is sight. Two qualities of Fire are brightness and reactivity, so it is no surprise that these people form the academics amongst us. Striking and noticeable eyes or a spark in the eye are common with this CEC. Fire has a quality of being oily, which can be noticed in Fire CEC's skin, which tends to be oily or reactive. In fact, Fiery people are quick to react, become frustrated easily, and are rapidly angered and irritated. Other common characteristics are being driven, sharp, and outspoken, and not letting things stand in their way. Life is lived at a fast pace and this can contribute to their hair going gray prematurely or to early death, as if they lived all their full life in a shorter timeframe.

Wind – Lom

Very Windy people might look as if they can be blown about in the wind. They are often "willowy," having fragile, slim frames with light bones. They are mostly either tall or small. Windy people often find it hard to be still, whether physically or mentally. They can be flighty, flaky, and accident-prone, and are sensitive both emotionally and physically. They can lack decisiveness because they can see things from both sides, yet they are full of ideas and are generally extremely creative, or completely devoid of creativity. They can excel at mathematics, languages, and computer work. As Windy people need to move a lot, they are often very active. Wind, as a light element, is closest to the spirit world and so Windy people are often hypersensitive to other realms, auras, ghosts, and so on. While it is easy for a Windy person to be knocked off balance, it is easy to bring them back to balance. This is because of the lightness of this element and the winds being able to blow both ways and change quickly.

A Personal Example of my Wind Imbalance

A while ago, I found myself thrown off balance by a particular situation. I was away from home and traveling most days, then coming home to an intimidating neighbor. Wind is a light element and in this instance I found I *quickly* became very scattered and lost my daily structure. I was shaky, with a racing heartbeat, and emotionally chaotic. I was on the edge and nervous, my mind was cluttered, and I was getting things wrong all the time. It became so extreme that I could not drive safely; I did not have the focus to concentrate and look at the road when I was driving. I was not able to action anything to help myself, as I was so flustered. If I had Fire as my CEC, I doubt this situation would have affected me in the same way. I would have been much more likely to get angry with the neighbor.

However, the neighbor moved out and this started calming the Winds. I could ground myself and feel safe at home. Being able to be at home more meant less travel and less movement, which also contributed to my Winds settling. These shifts had a massive impact on me, so much so that I could change a few daily habits and put some structure in place. I adjusted my diet a little to really help myself gain balance by eating lots of nuts and oily food (oil is very grounding and heavy, and highly beneficial for excited Wind element), made sure I slept at regular times, and meditated a lot. Once I had made these few adjustments, I *quickly* became balanced again.

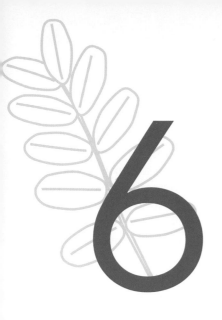

6

Physical Manifestations of Elements

Elements exist in various states, ranging from a healthy and balanced state of wellbeing, to being agitated, excited, weakened, broken, and missing (and more in between). When multiple elements are all unstable at the same time, this implies serious ill health. It is easiest to treat one unbalanced element. If it is left untreated, it will cause another element to be affected and this will continue, eventually having a spiraling effect on the others and causing dis-ease.

It is part of life that our health fluctuates, that we go through natural cycles, and that we experience suffering, pain, and disharmony. This is part of the human experience.

Here are some examples of weakened or agitated states, and how they would manifest differently in the body.

Earth

Earth is a solid and dense element. When this element is affected by disease, it means that the disease has reached such a point that it will be hard to reverse the progression. Additionally, Earth element can be damaged through accidents (for example, broken bones, cracked ribs, or torn ligaments), and despite the body having an amazing capacity to heal and function, there is often a weakness or irreparable damage left behind.

Loss of hair, weak hair, and rotting teeth suggest Earth in a weakened state. Weak or brittle bones, or organs that lack structural integrity (for example, weak lungs or bowel, or incontinence), are conditions where this element is weakened or below par. If the lungs are no longer functioning and breathing is difficult without machines, then the element is in more of a broken state.

Extra hair, bone spurs, and additional ribs, along with calcification of joints, tumors, fibroids, and cancer, show Earth element in an agitated or disturbed condition.

Water

Water is a slow and very cold element. Fluids more easily become stuck and stagnated, and so when Water is affected, the healing process can be slow. Water represents emotions such as worry, nostalgia, and depression, and these can also linger or move on slowly. People tend to feel the cold a lot, suffer from recurrent colds, are more likely to contract pneumonia, and have coughs that produce a lot of mucus rather than being dry. Someone with weakened Water element may have slow digestion or constipation, and hold on to toxins or fluids more easily.

In an agitated state, Water shows as an overproduction of sweat, an abundance of fluids (this could be mucus, saliva, or watery eyes, for example) and a tendency to retain water, and to have edema and puffy tissue. Agitated Water can also indicate conditions such as hypermobility, where there is excessive fluid collecting in a joint, urinary tract infections, edema, obesity, puffiness, and autism.

Weakened Water might show as lethargy, ignorance, or lack of understanding of other points of view. It could also present as low sex drive or stiff joints through lack of mobility (dried-up fluid in the joint capsule). Muscles that are atrophied indicate weakened Water, usually caused by lack of movement (Wind).

Fire

This element is responsible for our drive, passion, frustration, and anger. Fiery people are often easy to spot. It is a bit of a cliché but they might have red hair and freckles, or a reddish tone to their skin. Bright eyes, or sharp eyes and tongue, are most likely to indicate Fire element, as this is a sharp and reactive element. Fiery people tend to be the leaders among us, and can be bullies (even to themselves). They tend to be hotheads and are loud. They get the job done, make decisions quickly, and do not let anything stand in their way. This is the element of digestion, so Fire plays a large part in breaking down food. Excessive digestive Fire can mean that nutrients are not absorbed

properly, as they go through the body too rapidly. Hormones are linked to Fire, as it is the element of transformation. Notice how teenagers are suddenly angry and passionate about things; their hormones are stronger and sex is a driving force in those years, as is being career-driven. This is a particularly reactive time of life, but in a weakened state the opposite can be experienced: lack of drive and spark, lack of motivation, lack of warmth, poor digestion.

Agitated Fire would be seen with conditions such as acid reflux, cystitis, spots and rashes, inflammation, easy blushing, always being hot, easy burnout, rapid aging, early graying of the hair, early menstruation or menopause, or frequent fevers and high blood pressure.

Yet with weakened Fire you would notice someone's really cold skin, lacking the warmth of blood, very late hormonal development, low blood pressure, low libido, and no drive or passion.

Wind

Wind is the movement of branches on a tree and of the leaf falling to the ground. It is Wind that makes waves in the ocean and that brings the clouds and the rain in to the land. In the body it is *any* movement we make, whether that be birthing a baby, yawning, hiccupping, shaking, thinking, feeling, flexing our muscles, moving our eyes. It is Wind that moves blood and nutrients around our body and that moves food through our digestive tract, creates peristalsis, releases an egg in a woman's cycle, and makes sperm move.

All pain is attributed to Wind. The contraction of a muscle in spasm, a nerve pain, toothache, menstrual cramps, and any and all other pains are Wind element, the pain itself acting as a messenger and being the indicator. Nowadays, science tells us that all pain is in the brain and central nervous system, and if we see this through the lens of Thai medicine we know that the nerves are Sên, pathways through which there is movement.

With agitated Wind element we would see conditions such as dry skin, shaking, tremors, **Parkinson's disease**, restless leg syndrome, **Tourette's syndrome**, stammering, tics, general and shooting pains, lack of structure, anxiety, insomnia, over-thinking, tendency to boredom or over-stimulation, headaches, constipation, slow digestion, or slow circulation. Impeded movement, frozen shoulder, and numbness are indications of Wind in a weakened state.

It is also important to note that, for example, constipation could be attributed to depleted Water (to move it all through the digestive system), depleted Fire (low digestive fire to break things down), or weak Wind (not enough movement). We can see from this one example that it is difficult to be too prescriptive, and how Western diagnosis and terminology can be confusing. It is where consultations, diagnosis, experience, and study become important. Arthritis is another example of a Western label which is only partly useful if looking at the body through the Thai lens. This condition is mostly indictive of stiffness in the joint, with lack of movement and some inflammation/heat. The lack of movement is Wind element, the heat is Fire, and it could be that Water is also weakened.

> Side note: Keep in mind the fact that massage therapists are not officially allowed to diagnose, as we are not doctors. It is healthy to want to help people and to create treatments that are effective, but it is much safer to stay within your scope of practice and training.

However, once you undertake a course of study into any aspect of traditional medicine, you take on the responsibility to honor the lineage, the medicine, and the tradition. You are no longer a lay person; you have skills and knowledge that can help people.

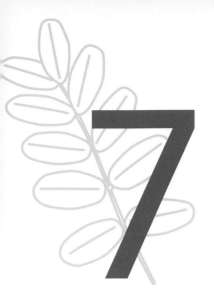

7

Dissection and Thai Anatomy

Dissection is a major theme running through this book because the experience of exploring inner space dramatically changed my view of life, and of my own body and human form.

The experience of seeing, touching, and connecting to the inner world of the body was a very spiritual and life-changing one.

Initially, I signed up to spend time in a cadaver lab to learn about anatomy in a way that no book could teach me. I felt I needed to see and feel the internal body to really understand it. However, what I discovered from the experience was that my perspective of the body, including my own, changed dramatically. In each cadaver I saw beauty and a reflection of my own body. I found that my practice soared, my hands had a heightened awareness as they touched the living, and my ability to teach and share the wonders of the body increased. Now, if students or clients ask me questions about the body, I have first-hand experiences that I can share with them and describe in detail.

Dissection also made me realize how accurately the textural layers of the body are noted in Thai anatomy. The practice of contemplating a corpse is one of the canonical meditations mentioned in the earliest Buddhist texts. I was amazed that before any Western dissections or autopsies were being recorded, the monks, practitioners, and **Reusi** had knowledge of the layers of the body, these same layers that I had been studying, palpating, and dissecting in the lab (Fig. 7.1).

Who are Reusi?

Reusi study natural and esoteric sciences. They are the Thai equivalent of **Yogis**, **Shamans**, and **Rishi** from other cultures. The Reusi all have different practices: some may focus their studies on meditation, others on mantras, planets, medicinal herbs, or the human form. They all study Buddha Dhamma, and additionally may also study **tantra**, astrology, **palmistry**, and other magical sciences. If herbs and medicine are their area, they will study each plant extensively, experimenting with ingesting it with or without food and meditating on the experience, feeling the effects it has on their body externally and internally. They record this information and are able to pass it on to benefit others.

Chapter 7

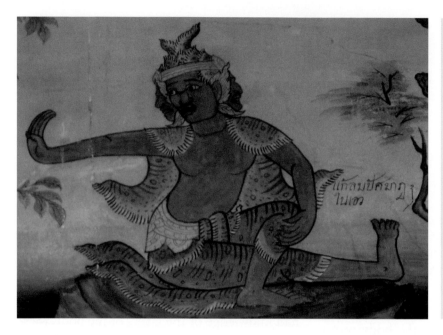

In the past, the Reusi also experimented with their own bodies through self-massage, stretching, movement, and breath. From this practice, they adapted the self-care system (Reusi Dat Ton), later to become what we now know as Thai bodywork.

As in the UK, where dissection of any bodies other than those of murderers was illegal until the nineteenth century, it is likely that in Thailand there may have been religious rules or taboos about cutting human flesh. Sometimes, people would leave their bodies to the **Sangha** (community), with the sole intention of it being studied, in much the same way that people leave their bodies to science nowadays.

When people died, if they were not able to afford to be burned or buried, they would have been eaten by jackals, dogs, or vultures. The monks and Reusi would have learned about the body from observing this process as the body disintegrated to the ethers (Fig. 7.2). This process must have been profoundly interesting, yet not for the faint-hearted. I can only imagine the putrefaction that would take place in the tropical heat and the dispersal of layers being eaten from the inside by bugs, larvae, and bacteria.

There is a practice where monks and Reusi meditate on the decomposing bodies with a strong focus on the elements of the body dispersing, to improve their knowledge and understanding of the body. This practice dates back to the time of the Buddha and is still in existence now. In doing this, they were able to see the internal landscape of the body, the structures and layers in situ, and could contemplate their functions, textures, and disease causation, much as in the cadaver lab. In my own quest to find similar answers I have stared death in the face many times during

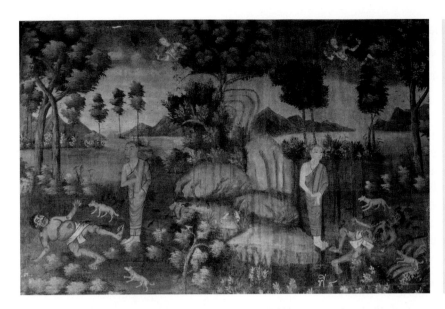

Fig. 7.2
A mural from a temple wall in Thailand, of monks contemplating corpses as they begin decomposing. With kind permission of Tim Bewer.

dissection. I often find myself thinking about and having huge reverence for the lengths the Reusi went to in their quest to understand human form and to share their knowledge with lay people and help heal others, something I also see in modern-day times with fellow **Somanauts**.

During dissection, there is a tangible energy in the room that is completely unlike anything I have ever experienced before and that changes as the layers are **reflected**. It is busy in the lab: there are lots of projects and explorations going on and it is easy to lose oneself in timeless focus. However, it does affect the nervous system, and good teachers will make sure there is time to delve into the feelings and effects that the experience produces. It is emotional, humbling, and deeply life-affirming, and gives so much to be thankful for. I say this because the process of dissection in a lab, guided by teachers, is a mind-altering spiritual experience which cannot be too dissimilar to the experiences of the Reusi.

Anatomical Layers

One of the foundations of Thai anatomy is to recognize and acknowledge anatomical layers, and to absorb the importance of treating them from superficial to deep. Each layer has a different texture, and there are patterns in the body that can be seen repeating over and over again.

During the type of dissection I have participated in, led by my teachers, Gil Hedley and Julian Baker, we spend time acknowledging continuity, as well as touching and palpating internal textures and structures at the superficial level. Once we have studied these to our satisfaction, within the time constraints that we are under, we remove that layer and repeat the process, going deeper to the next layer. When we reach the visceral layer, the focus becomes the organs and the Sên (pathways of movement in the body, such as lymph, tendons, nerves, and vessels) that carry nutrients, waste, blood, and messages, as well as the spine and brain.

Chapter 7

"By their textures ye shall know them!"

Gil Hedley, personal communication, 2014

When we perform traditional Thai bodywork in a treatment, each of the layers is cared for and addressed. Many techniques are applied – some with tools, some with hands – so that skin, superficial and deep fasciae, muscle, nerves, tendons, ligaments, bone, and viscera are all nourished, balanced, supported, cared for, and dealt with. Treating in this way is safe for the body and provides the most effective approach. I believe that the most therapeutic of touches are enfolded in this approach, and that anything else is a bombardment on the body.

Side note: Think of the body as that person's home. With bodywork, we should knock politely at the door and wait to be admitted, rather than rudely barge or break in.

Through the dissection process, one starts to see the internal and external worlds reflecting each other as a mirror image. Internally, we have vessels and nerves that, when we look at the whole body, resemble trees. Internal textures and patterns are mirrored in the world around us: stripes, honeycombs, and spirals. Superficial fascia is like sponge from the seabed; we have blood running through our veins like water running through rivers. A structure that lies within our abdomen made of **mesentery** and intestine perfectly resembles a bouquet of flowers when lifted out and kept attached at its root. Muscles look like ploughed fields. There are cavernous, curious spaces.

Nothing is separate: every single time you touch, move, or press the body, communication is happening, a touch response is being activated, affecting Wind element (otherwise known as movement) throughout the whole. In Thai massage and bodywork we acknowledge layers, but I encourage you to consider that these layers do not only run from superficial to deep, but are also whole-body continuations.

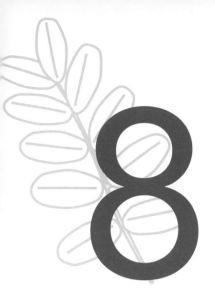

8 The Five Textural Layers

When we look at a body, how often do we bring our attention to the **morphology** that is being presented into the space which that person takes up?

Not often, and yet it provides useful information that can tell us a lot about that person. Is it primarily the superficial fascia we see shaping the space around them? Perhaps the bony layer is the most prominent layer defining the shape. Is it the muscle layer that shapes the space or do you see the visceral layer, with the guts protruding?

Earth and Water elements make up the physical body in Thai anatomy.

The five layers of the body (their structure, not their function) are all Earth element body parts. Any fluids associated with the body are Water element. Skin is a good example, as it provides resistance and support (Earth element function), yet its malleability has Water element quality. Skin without Water element would be hard and inflexible. Additionally, Water element is also cohesive: it binds and sticks things together.

Thai anatomy acknowledges five layers of the body, and it is these layers that are recognized in hands-on treatments. There are, of course,

more layers in the body: for example, the skin can be separated into many layers beyond the **epidermal** and **dermal**. There are two obvious layers of fascia (superficial and deep), which can be separated further (with the right tools) into many more layers in dissection.

The layers of the body are:

1. skin

2. fascia, muscle, and soft tissue

3. channels/Sên

4. bone/joints

5. viscera/organs.

The layer model comes from monks having watched a body decomposing (see Fig. 7.2) but it is likely that what was seen was a density, a depth with various textures and qualities, from superficial to deep. The layer model is a teaching tool that is used for hands-on application of touch, rather than an accurate description of anatomy, which is far more complex than this.

All components of the body interconnect with, and are interdependent on, each other; none works in isolation. In its innate and infinite wisdom, the body detects subtle changes, which ripple through and are experienced by the whole organism. Every input of touch affects every part of the mind, body, and soul, as nothing is separate and there are no "parts" of the body that work in isolation.

When applying manual therapeutic techniques to the body, it helps to have a clear understanding of the layers being touched and the far-reaching effects on all workings of the body.

The layer model is important for the therapist because it is a way of working with integrity and allows the practitioner to ease deeper into the recipient's body as it relaxes. However, the body has a network of fascia that has astonishing intelligence and is multi-directional and multi-dimensional. It communicates throughout the whole in all directions, through all the layers, through all dimensions and angles. (This is depicted in Thai medicine as the Winds moving through the Sên and explains why you can press a point in one area and feel its effects in another.)

In a lab, each "layer" that is differentiated can be distinguished by texture.

Dissection teacher Gil Hedley has given each layer a textural description and that is what I use here.

First Layer – Skin: "Wetsuit"

"The skin is the outer surface of the brain, or the brain is the deepest layer of the skin."

Deane Juhan, 2003

Skin is the largest organ of the body and is the superficial representation of the nervous system. It has thousands of nerve endings and neural offshoots embedded within it.

It is a fascinating structure. It is colorful, self-heals, is sensual and perceptive, and is in constant communication with the whole body. Skin has tiny fibers that root firmly to the superficial fascia, so that they tightly adhere to each other. The only tool that can differentiate one from the other is a very sharp **scalpel**. A proficient hand is needed to carry out this separation. When we touch this layer with our hands, we touch the *whole* body and *all* its layers; the whole body responds.

The skin is rich in nerve endings and capillaries, extensions of the nerve and heart trees. This means that the lightest touch has an immediate physiological impact on life-sustaining systems, and instigates rest and repair through the parasympathetic nervous system.

The skin layer has many functions: it protects, cushions, regulates, and eliminates. The skin is made of multiple layers, as well having different textures that can be observed and palpated superficially (smooth, soft, hard, rough, dry, oily, spotty, bumpy – to name but a few). It can be hot or cold, sweaty or clammy, and highly sensitive or numb to the touch.

We are generally familiar with the texture of skin. We can easily see it; we know its typical consistency. In some ways, this makes it a layer we do not give much thought to. But if we look more deeply, we see it as a revealing and expressive organ that is affected by emotions and mood. Emotional responses, such as blushing with embarrassment or going pale with fright, are beyond our conscious control.

These are examples of how we lay ourselves bare, showing our heart via the vessels of the circulatory system to the skin. In Thai medicine, the heat rising to the face or the pallor that comes with fright would be Fire element, the Fire of emotion in agitated and weakened states.

The skin is always the first layer that needs to be taken care of when giving a Thai massage.

Second Layer – Fascia, Muscle, and Soft Tissue

Superficial Fascia: "Spongy Bodysuit"

Superficial fascia, or the **hypodermis**, is the layer directly below and intimately attached to the many layers of skin. It is a whole-body coating, with a visually sponge-like, bouncy, and soft texture; this layer of adipose tissue is incredibly strong and constitutes a malleable and structured fluid component of the body. While the superficial fascia might look spongy, it has strength to it that a sponge does not.

The superficial fascia has fibrous connections and globular textures. The lobules are pressed together in a disordered but repeated pattern, and have **perifascia** (connective tissue) in each of them. This loose, areolar connective tissue is found all over the body, from the fat around the heart, lungs, and other vital organs to the eyeballs, genitals, and adrenal glands (Fig. 8.1). It has a vibrational intelligence, and is able to communicate and receive information like a highly perceptive antenna.

The superficial fascia distinguishes male and female body shapes; it is primarily a whole-body protection, a bit like bubble wrap, and is made of loose areolar tissue and fat cells. It is a lymphoid, endocrinal, and metabolic organ that is an essential part of the whole. It has various depths and is a sensory, sensual organ.

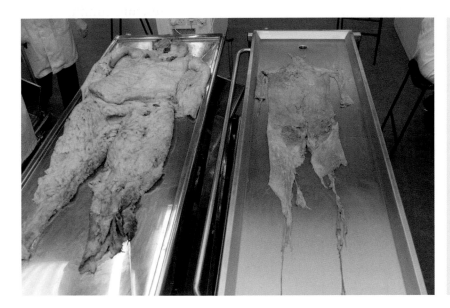

Fig. 8.1
The superficial fascia dissected with continuity from two very different-shaped bodies. By special permission of Functional Fascia.

Chapter 8

This layer is more familiar than we may initially realize, for it is what we feel and touch when we massage. It is the soft, fleshy, springy texture that we feel when we hug, squeeze, or come into contact with someone; it is the flesh on our belly, legs, arms, and buttocks, as well as the thinner flesh we find in areas such as the face, back of the hands and top of the feet. This is often a much-hated, ridiculed, focused-on layer of the body, a layer that exposes and expresses vulnerabilities, and can be cut out or got rid of. It is a layer that (in the Western world) is considered to be cuddly and cute in the young, but commonly rejected in adults. It can even be fashionable. It is a layer that can be soft, malleable, and plentiful, or incredibly thin like paper. In other areas of the world, this layer is seen very differently: it portrays wealth, and the more there is of it, the more beautiful one is perceived to be.

Sadly, this layer receives a lot of press and attention but for negative reasons, rather than for being the fundamental, protective, intrinsic layer that it is.

Gil Hedley beautifully describes this layer:

"It is a sensory system, a metabolic regulator, an insulator, an organ of emotional expression, an organ of sensuality and sexuality, a resource, a protection, a comfort."

Gil Hedley, personal correspondence, 2016

This makes me wonder why we do not have much more appreciation of all its wonderful functions.

This layer is Earth element; it offers resistance and support, but has a high fluid content – hence the sponge-like texture and pliability.

Gil Hedley also called this membranous layer the "filmy fascia," which describes, brilliantly and simply, the exact texture of the epimysium, a gliding, sliding layer that strongly resembles Saran wrap (cling film). He more recently renamed it the perifascia. To experience it in your own body, you can wrap your hand around your forearm, grasping it. Now maintain that hold, keep your arm still, and move the skin up and down – as you do this, you will be feeling the layers in your grasp sliding over the filmy fascia. Nerves and vessels are wrapped in their own perifascia, and glide over and under deep fascia via this filmy membranous and elastic fascial layer.

This membranous layer, found all over the body, allows for differential movement between two layers in the musculo-skeletal system. It is collagenous, slippery, and elastic (Fig. 8.2). There are a few areas in the body that do not have perifascia, such as the hands and feet (we do not really need these areas of our body to have sliding surfaces) and the abdomen (which has a specialized **serous fluid**).

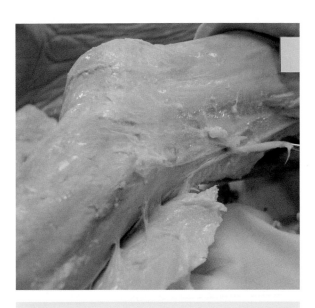

Fig. 8.2
The perifascia and deep fascia sheath around the knee and tibia. By kind permission of Functional Fascia.

Dense, Deep Fasciae: "Strappy Rubber Bands"

All fascia is the fabric of us – it holds us together and forms an intricate and complex communicating network that provides structure. If we stood all the bones of our skeleton upright without any support, they would fall to the ground and land in a heap.

The deeper fascia ranges in thickness, depending on its job in the body. It has a multi-layered, cross-fibered, and strappy tissue texture. It is both stabilizing and flexible, and surrounds and supports the muscles. In some areas it is anchored. Its density is variable.

In places, such as the ilio-tibial band on the lateral side of the leg, it is particularly thick, wide, and fibrous. So is the plantar fascia on the underside of the foot, and both are often termed "**aponeurosis**" due to their band-like similarity to tendons.

From the end of the first month in utero, fascia is already forming and is part of the embryological make-up. All organs and tissue in the body develop from three layers of cells: the **endoderm**, **mesoderm**, and **ectoderm**. Connective tissue is produced by the mesoderm, which also produces our muscles and bones.

The levels of hydration in the body are reflected in the health of soft tissue. Our bodies are made up of a high percentage of water, and a large proportion of this is stored in the connective tissue.

"Your fascia is a body wide storehouse for much of this water, both inside its cells and soaking throughout its fibrous threads. This extracellular fascial fluid flows between the cells and fibers of your fascial 'wetsuit' … fascia relies on liquidity for proper cellular function and replication. When we do not move enough or address ongoing poor postural habits, the fascia starts to lose its ability to absorb fluid easily and then becomes dehydrated. Movement hydrates the body internally."

Jill Miller, 2014

Chapter 8

The network of fascia, made up primarily of collagen and lipids, continues to be laid down in the body until about twenty-four years of age. This internal fabric changes, depending on what is needed for optimum movement, strength, and mobility.

Each person's body is unique, partly due to the various things we do when we perform different tasks, including how we move, express, accept, and nourish ourselves.

For example, when we sit, repeatedly looking down at our phones, our fascia will eventually start to respond to this pattern of behavior. It will start laying down fibrous tissue in its attempt to help support and maintain this position. If we keep looking at our phones in the same position over many long hours, over months the fascia starts to get more fibrous, toughening in places like the nape of the neck, which makes it harder to move. This causes discomfort and means we have decreased range of movement, most often leading to a diminished ability to move through natural ranges because it causes discomfort.

Side note: Ideally, we would use Reusi Dat Ton to re-educate the body through movement, breath, and self-massage, and Thai manual therapy for passive movement and therapeutic touch techniques.

Everything is wrapped in fascia: muscles (which have fascia interpenetrating and surrounding them), tendons, ligaments, the membranes around the brain, spinal cord or nerves, and the bags that hold each organ.

"In all of these linings, wrappings, cables and moorings [connective tissue] is a continuous substance and every single part of the body is connected to every other part by virtue of its network; every part of us is in its embrace."

Deane Juhan, 2003

Muscle

Once the superficial, filmy, and deep fasciae have been removed from the body in dissection and the muscles are exposed, we can clearly see their familiar striations and meaty texture. But without the fabric holding them together, they spill out and have an uncontained look to them. This reveals a vulnerability; they are no longer protected or held in place by their supporting structure and network.

Skeletal muscles are well-organized tissues spiraling around the body in one whole-body continuation, with perifascia and neurovasculature surrounding and weaving their way through and around them. Often, the muscle blends flawlessly into the fascia, where it disappears and becomes another structure. On a physical level, muscles are able to be contractile and expansive; they can be manipulated by force and will to be more clearly defined. On an emotional level, they are "an organ of will and emotive expression," says Gil Hedley.

In Thai bodywork we work on releasing bound-up tissue to make it more pliable in order to be able to work on the channels and Sên to effect physiological change in the body.

Not all muscles have the clear definition of a membrane between them but continue from one to the next. Examples of this are the **piriformis** and gluteus medius.

Side note: Not all muscles are striated; there are smooth muscles in the body, found, for example, within the walls of the stomach, intestines, and ureter. They contract involuntarily.

The psoas muscles

It seems important to briefly mention the psoas muscles (iliopsoas, psoas major, and psoas minor), which are long, deep muscles that emerge from either side of the thoracic spine and travel down to the lumbar spine. The psoas minor eventually becomes a thin tendon at the pelvis and the psoas major travels through the pelvis and over the hip bone, blending seamlessly into the lesser trochanter. It forms a triangular shape right at the center of the body.

I hear many people talk about the psoas and, as the only muscle that attaches the upper and lower body, it is significant. Having dissected the body and looked into this on each cadaver, I have seen that it is not possible to actually touch the psoas with our hands in massage or bodywork. It is too deep and there are too many other structures in the way. However, with touch, we can still affect this muscle because all touch has the ability to impact the deeper layers, and when there is a movement of Wind through the body (from superficial to deep, or from one place to another), there is a physiological impact.

Being the only muscle that attaches the upper and lower body has far-reaching implications on a physical, structural, and functional level. This muscle is not the only one to contract as part of the fear response, but it does travel in close proximity to the heart, diaphragm, and solar plexus, not to mention how it brushes against other viscera on its journey to the lower limbs. Hence, for all these reasons, the psoas is often described as a "muscle of emotional expression," although the whole body is continually expressing emotion, which we can see clearly through posture, gait, and function. If we think about this on an energetic level, this muscle grows from the spine and develops early in utero; it is often called a "core muscle." While our body is one whole, continuous, tidal organism that cannot be separated into parts, the fact that this muscle is one of the first to give support alludes to it having more "depth" to it than a superficial muscle. The psoas has a close relationship with the adrenal glands and is thought to contract under emotional stress, readying us for fight or flight. Another description for this structure is a "muscle of the soul" (Liz Koch, 2012), as it is so deep, long, and old, and plays a vital role as connector.

The heart, diaphragm, and lungs are neighbors to this muscle and they also share the perifascial sheath; because of this, they have a synergistic and differential relationship. The contraction and expansion of the psoas, and the state it is in – whether holding on or letting go, influences the breath, in the same way that the breath in turn influences this muscle and many other structures, tissues, and cells in the body. The psoas, having formed early in utero, might have a significant impact on our posture, on how we hold ourselves and express ourselves, and on the parasympathetic nervous system.

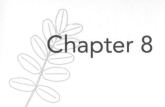

Chapter 8

Third Layer – Channels/Sên

The continuation of fascia in the musculo-skeletal framework separates muscles and is found between muscle and bone. When we are palpating the body, these areas have more give. They feel like places of space, or potential space, that can be sunk into and are areas to which a therapist's hands are often drawn. In a healthy and well-hydrated body they may also feel more fluid-like, with a less dense texture than would be encountered if pressing straight on to a muscle. The channels are places that facilitate deeper entry into the body, where the practitioner can stimulate the underlying Sên.

So, What Are Sên?

The Sên (see Chapter 10) are very tangible structures like nerves, tendons, lymph vessels, blood vessels, and ligaments. They are pathways that facilitate movement such as blood flow, fluid exchange, communication, thought processes, waste removal, and so on.

On a micro level, they also permit movements that occur in the body and that we know happen, but are too small to see, like the circulation of hormones, cellular activity, the action of digestive enzymes, and activity along neural pathways.

Thought and emotions are also acknowledged as pathways of movement and are identified as the subtle Sên. They are movements that we cannot initially see but which we experience. Like all thought or emotional processes, they become physical as they slow down and become form. If you take a moment to observe the posture of someone who is happy compared with that of someone who is depressed, what do you notice? Do you see

how their whole body and their movements express their internal and hidden self? Are they hunched at the shoulders to protect their hearts?

By pressing the channels, the practitioner activates (gives touch input to) the (deeper) Sên. If the soft tissue is stuck and bound up, and there is not much differential movement, the practitioner uses manual therapy techniques to soften and hydrate them, to make them more malleable so as not to bully a way into the body by going to the deeper layers without respecting the tissues. The input of pressing into these channels becomes like lighting a spark, igniting communication to the deeper underlying structures.

The depth of Sên varies, depending on the area of the body. For example, on the top of the foot the channels and underlying Sên are superficial, in comparison to the channels between the hamstrings which are located deeper in the body, requiring an adjustment of pressure to reach them. If we look at the Achilles tendon as a pathway of movement, the channels sit on either side of it (lateral and medial to it).

Fourth Layer – Bone/Joints

As well as the soft tissues, which we have previously discussed, connective tissue is now considered by anatomists to be both blood and lymph (fluid tissue), and cartilage and bone (hard tissue). Bone, with its dense, crystalized collagen structure, is developed at the mesodermal stage in the embryo. Like all other fascia, bone has an ability to heal and regenerate. Wolff's law of remodeling, a theory developed in 1892, describes the following in relation to the forces put upon

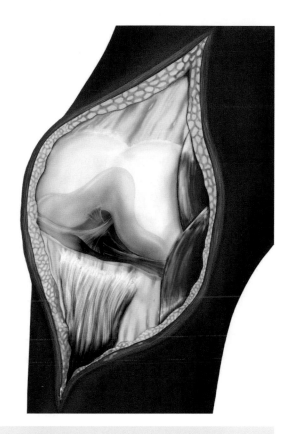

Fig. 8.3
The knee joint and synovial fluid.

bone: "bone changes its external shape and internal (**cancellous**) architecture in response to stresses acting on it."

The bone layer, while mainly referring to the joints in the body (Fig. 8.3), also protects vital organs (ribcage) and supports the organs of the body (pelvic basin).

This layer of the body is mainly addressed by working with range of motion of a joint, traction, and vibrational techniques.

It is also used in bodywork by the therapist to apply deep pressure, often using knees, ulna, side of foot, knuckles, shins, lateral and medial epicondyles (elbow), and calcaneus (heel).

Fifth Layer – Viscera/Organs

We experience our organs very lightly, despite their huge and heavy mass. There are pressure differentials in the body that hold organs in place and keep them below the diaphragm. In Thai medicine, the organization of these organs is attributed to Kwan, which is best described as an organizing life-force energy of the whole body, and of the individual organs. Kwan is how our organs know how to stay in position. However, posture and life habits can defeat the natural weightless ease of the organs in situ (see Chapter 16).

This is a profoundly intelligent area of the body, the body center that relates and communicates to the whole. It is a rich and abundant place, where many Sên are located. These include the gross Sên (abdominal aorta), as well as the minor (arteries, nerves, and so on), the invisible (digestive enzymes), and the subtle (emotional or gut instinct pathways of communication). The arrangement of viscera is exquisite and each person has a unique visceral beauty that distinguishes them as individuals, like a second face.

Layer Model

The layer model is a story of the body, a map that allows us to form clear intentions as to where and what is being worked on. But in reality, each layer to which touch input is applied will work on every layer, part, and continuation of the body. Everything is made out of everything else: a tendon becomes the fascial sac around a muscle, which then interweaves with another muscle before wrapping around an organ and diving deeper into the body in a spiral shape. There is blood in bone. There is movement in muscle tissue. Not all movement is related to Sên. Sên are primary pathways of movement in the body. Think of the tiny vessels, capillaries, and invisible Sên when you are next working on the skin. When you are working on the muscle, fat, and tissue layer, remember that there are also invisible Sên and minor Sên, so each technique you use will be addressing Sên. When you work on bone, you are working on Sên, as it is a physical pathway of movement in the body.

Side note: Sên are *primary pathways* of movement but not all movement is Sên. Remember that Sên are always structures shaped like noodles, hair, strands, or wire. A muscle moves and a bone moves, as does the blood inside them. There is also movement in the body that is not Sên-related, such as the passage of food through the digestive tract, the movement of limbs when walking, the fluid movement of the heart, and the expansion and contraction of the lungs.

9

Thai Medicine: The Five Roots

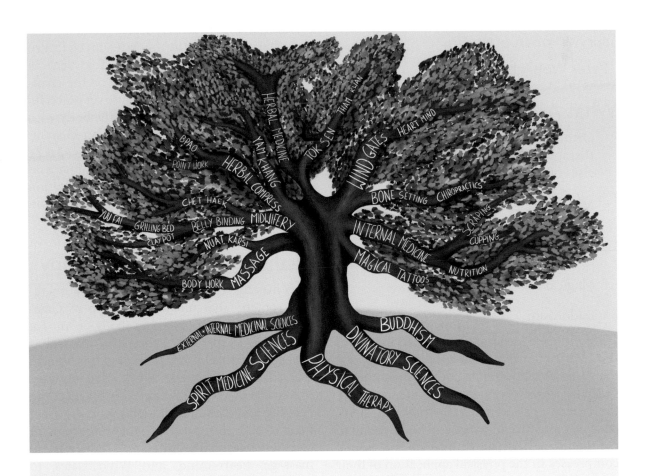

Fig. 9.1
The five roots of Thai medicine.

Chapter 9

We can use the simple analogy of a tree when we talk about the Thai medicine system (Fig. 9.1). The practice is like a mature and powerful tree, one with strong roots that feed the trunk, which in turn gives life to the big and small branches, and leaves, flowers, and fruit. It is these ancient, interconnected roots that give life to the medicine. No one root feeds the trunk in isolation for they all work interdependently to nourish the whole tree.

> "It is the root that looks after the survival of an organism."

Peter Wohlleben, 2017

What Are the Five Roots?

- Orthopedic sciences: external, physical therapy, which includes the physical exercises of Reusi Dat Ton.

- Medical sciences: internal therapies and herbal medicine.

- Divinatory sciences.

- Magical sciences.

- Buddhism.

Practitioners generally specialize in one of the five roots, or a branch of that root, but their knowledge extends beyond their chosen specialty, interweaving with some or all of the others. For example, Thai physical therapists who practice massage and bodywork will use medicinal balms, liniments, and herbal compresses in the physical application of their work, but these come from the medical sciences root. They implement knowledge and use products from this root, as they are formulas that aid healing. Some practitioners make medicinal balms, often being given formulas by their teachers or other practitioners to use in their practice. Physical therapy specialists also make herbal infusions, decoctions, and formulas for their clients to ingest to support the physical work internally. If their level of training allows, they may also suggest healing foods that nourish and support the body internally, often based on elemental imbalance.

Additionally, they may learn therapies that are physical by nature but are, in fact, also spirit medicine: for example, **Tok Sên**, in which a mallet and peg are used on the channels to stimulate Sên. It is a gentle yet powerful technique that works deep into the body with vibration, while at the same time an incantation is silently repeated. Practitioners must be initiated in the practice of this technique and their tools are blessed with a magic incantation for extra healing powers. Tok Sên comes from the **Lanna** tradition in Northern Thailand.

Orthopedic/Physical Therapy

Thai massage comes under the external therapies root of Thai medicine, known as **Gaia-Ya-Bam-Bat** (*Gaia* meaning body, *bam bat* translating as therapy). While Thai massage is probably the best known therapy in this branch, there are many others, which Thai massage practitioners may utilize in their practice: **fire cupping** and **Khuut**, **blood-letting** (to draw out toxic blood), chiropractic (bone setting), point and Sên release therapy, scarf work, visceral massage, heart–mind, and Wind Gates, to name but a few. (You can read more about these techniques and others in Chapter 20.)

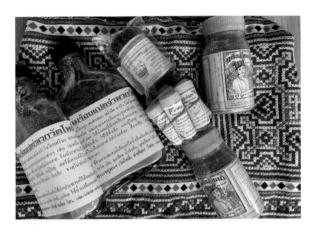

Fig. 9.2
Generic herbal Lanna and Thai medicine formulas for internal use.

Internal/herbal Medicine

This root of Thai medicine includes the prescription of single herbs and herbal formulas, using plants, berries, seeds, leaves, roots, and animal products such as the gall bladder or kidneys (Fig. 9.2). In this root you will find anything from wound care and bone healing to dietary counselling and herbal medicine.

When there is an imbalance, food is prescribed to rebalance and nourish the elements of the body. Nutritional advice is given and daily eating habits are looked at. When herbs are used singly, they fall under a nine-**taste system** category, but when foods are used as medicine they are organized into a six-taste system. There is also a further four-taste system that correlates to the external application of herbs.

Side note: Taste systems are categorized as sweet, salty, spicy, pungent, astringent, bitter, aromatic, and so on. (Read more about this in Chapter 15.)

Practitioners of this specialty who work with all taste systems may also prepare and use balms, liniments, and compresses externally as a method to get herbs into the body. For example, if a patient has a joint problem, they might be given a herbal formula to ingest, but if they are in pain, the herbs to use with physical therapy would be indicated.

Divinatory Sciences

This root involves the practitioners having great insight and intuition, as well as in-depth knowledge and studies of astrology, palmistry, **numerology**, **geomancy**, Tarot, and more. These are used to diagnose, gain insight about, and treat current illness and elemental constitution, as well as understanding the elemental predisposition to diseases and imbalances that may come into being in the future.

This branch of Thai medicine also correlates in specific ways to the element system. For example, each of the four fingers and the thumb represents an element, and the signs of the Zodiac (determined at conception, not birth) correspond to seasonal elemental associations and planetary influences.

The day and time of your birth, place of birth, and the planetary alignments and formations all have significance. The day of birth has meaning, as it can decipher

characteristics, relationships, and natural inclinations in the same way that those in the West view astrological signs.

Side note: In Thailand, each day of the week is aligned with a specific posture of the Buddha, apart from Wednesday, when there is a morning and evening Buddha. The postures are seated, with hands folded or held out in front, reclining, or meditational.

In Thailand, there is a strong belief in the world of spirits, ghosts, and deities. Magical sciences practitioners perform Shamanic, ritualistic magic practices for healing, protection, and guidance, and to dispel spirits that are causing harm and ill health.

Magical Sciences

Spirits feature heavily in Thai culture and are often seen to cause imbalances and disrupt health.

There are many traditions found in this root, some of which also include the use of herbs to work on the body and drive out spirits that might be causing harm. Many healing practices and tools are used in this root, which include incantations, mantras, **amulets**, hot coals, deities, spiritual tattoos called **Sak Yan**, and many more. Some practices involve blowing sacred words on to the body, called **Bpao**. Another uses an egg to drive out toxins and evil from the body.

With magical sciences, we can see how the aforementioned roots can be interwoven with this one. A Lanna technique called **Chet** might be used by a physical therapist, herbal medicine practitioner, or magic medicine practitioner. It involves applying feather-light touch with a piece of **plai** root or a medicinal leaf to wipe or stroke the body to draw out impurities, and is a clear example of herbal, physical, and magic medicinal practices combined.

Another practice that involves all three of these roots is one in which heat from coals, combined with medicinal oils, is applied to the body. The practitioner first wets their heel in the medicinal oil, before dipping the oily heel into the fire and then using it to rub the recipient's body to drive out spirits. This practice is also linked to the transformational element of Fire.

Side note: Traditionally, it is only male practitioners who can perform this particular treatment. This is to protect women from spirits, as they are seen to be more easily affected by them, especially around the time of menarche.

Spirits can easily be agitated, so it is part of Thai culture to look after them, keep them happy, acknowledge, and honor them; even so, they can still cause trouble and harm. This branch of Thai medicine deals with problems caused by the spirit world that affect the body (manifesting as depletion of essence, illness, strange behavior, and more). The mind and life-force (Kwan) of an individual also have the ability to be affected by spirits.

Elementally, someone with Wind as their core element constitution (CEC; see Chapter 5), especially if they have a Wind imbalance, is more easily affected by the spirit world because

Wind is the lightest element. But anyone, no matter what their core element, can be affected by spirits. Black magic, malevolence, wrongdoing, or disruption to land or a house are all possible causes and there are many more.

Sak Yan is the practice of magical tattooing. A practitioner is initiated into this tradition and studies Buddha Dhamma. Incantations and mantras are quietly spoken or silently/mentally repeated throughout the process of tattooing, which imbues the tattoo with magic. Traditionally, medicinal herbs are used in the ink and have healing properties. The design of the Yan is related to astrological readings and is primarily for protection or attraction; they also commonly feature images that represent the Buddha, who symbolizes the path of enlightenment.

While it is not imperative for a Thai massage practitioner to be Buddhist, it is essential to acknowledge that Thai medicine *is* Buddhist medicine and to see how intricately it is woven throughout and feeds all the roots of this medical system.

Buddhism

This is the fifth root of Thai medicine and it permeates the system. It is the basis for the rules of being a practitioner, for the theory of medicine and the elements. Buddhism is predominantly a philosophy for life. It is the mental health root of Thai medicine due to its focus on meditation and other practices for cultivating a more peaceful mind.

The Buddha is seen as the ultimate healer. He was born into the warrior caste as a prince. Years before his birth, it was predicted that he would become either a great spiritual leader or a great king. He initially led a very sheltered and privileged life under the protection of his parents, who wanted to keep him from all the unpleasant aspects of normal life. Yet it was impossible for him to be protected all the time. At one point he left the compound where he lived with his wife and child, and he saw the reality of life for local people.

He witnessed suffering, sickness, old age, and death. He also saw a wandering ascetic, who had renounced the material world, walking peacefully along the road with an alms bowl. He felt drawn to discovering deeper meaning in his own life and so he decided to leave the compound and find ways to ease and understand all suffering in the world. This became his predominant focus, his life's work. He devised certain formulas that are prescriptions for leading a harmonious life, recipes for happiness and balance. Initially, he lived as an ascetic for a few years with seven other ascetics, who later became the first of his disciples and who would form the first Sangha, carrying on his teachings.

Suttas are literature defining the teachings of the Buddha, called Buddha Dhamma. There are many, which can be found in the **Pali** Canon, and they include the noble eight-fold path, eight worldly concerns, five precepts, three universal truths, and four noble truths. They are profound philosophical lessons.

The mind can easily cause suffering that affects every aspect of life, often becoming physical pain, and that can lead to imbalance throughout one's life. Techniques such as meditation help create space in the mind and provide stable mental health. The regular practice of meditation brings awareness, calm, and attention to experience.

The symbolism of numbers is another instance of how Buddhism contributes to Thai medicine. An example is the number 108, which is symbolic of the 108 Winds in the body, and the number of beads on a Jap **mala** (a set of beads in the form of a necklace) used in meditation or mantra; it also signifies 108 feelings. The number 5 relates to the five elements, five directions, five limbs (the two legs, the two arms and the head, which is classified as the fifth limb), and five Buddhas (there have been four until now and there will eventually be another in years to come, when the teachings of the current Buddha are no longer practiced). The number 8 is significant, as it correlates to the noble eight-fold path (a Buddhist teaching that leads to a better and more harmonious life).

Side note: We have six incoming senses (smell, touch, taste, sound, vision, and what the mind perceives). There are three sensations (pleasant, unpleasant, and neutral). We experience the world through the past, present, and future.

10

Sên and Channels

In this chapter I want to redress past inaccuracies and clarify Sên as pathways of movement (Fig. 10.1). I spent many years practicing Thai massage on the premise that Sên were "energy lines" and that I was predominantly working with the energy flow in the body.

I then went on to teach Sên within this context but there were big doubts in my mind. I could not quite understand how this concept and theory of Sên were actually Thai. Furthermore, it was proving difficult to find information about Thai theory, and my need for clarity about Sên was increasing. There was something important missing, but at that time I did not know what.

In fact, there was so little Thai theory available, despite traveling to Thailand, searching bookshops, and later on using the internet for research. Information was scarce and anything I could find was about Ayurveda theory, Chinese philosophy, or yoga. There were lots of Thai massage books with various combinations of stretches and sequences, but no explanation of a theory to back it all up. It was as if the practice was the theory.

In my classroom, I was observing how hard some students were finding the Sên work, fumbling around trying to locate the "energy lines," develop a feeling for them, and experience the flow of energy. They were working with eyes closed, tuning in and really concentrating, but then feeling disheartened when they were not able to *feel* the energy. It was an area of the work that they least enjoyed performing. Conversely, clients found the experience of the thumb press technique very beneficial physically.

When I finally discovered that there is, in fact, a whole system of Thai medicine, it was transformative. Understanding Sên from the perspective of traditional medicine altered my practice dramatically, and I also saw a huge change in the competency of students studying the bodywork.

Side note: These inaccuracies are still being taught the world over, Thailand included. They are standardized, Westernized, and corrupted, and show no relevance to Sên as they are written about in traditional medical texts.

Sên in Traditional Theory

In traditional Thai medicine, Sên are physical structures in the body that are listed as an

Chapter 10

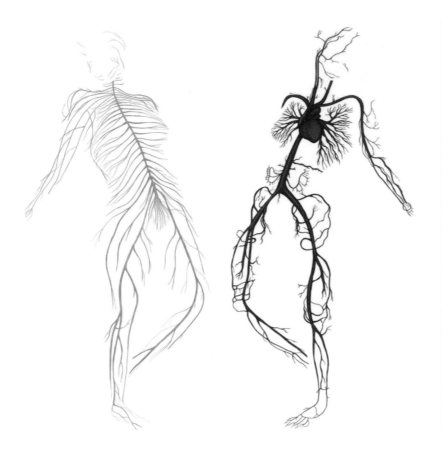

Fig. 10.1
Sên trees: path-
ways of movement
through vessels
and nerves, both of
which are Sên.

Earth element body part (of which there are twenty). As per Thai element theory, all things with an experience of solidity and whose function provides support and resistance are exhibiting Earth element. When I talk about Sên in relation to Earth element, I am referring to their *actual* gross structure: that is, the fabric of which they are made. As Earth is one of the tangible elements that make up the gross anatomy of the body (Water being the other), it should be clear that, when working with Sên, we are working with the most palpable part of the body. Working on the physical body is much more familiar than working with energy. This leads students and practitioners

to be more comfortable and competent in this realm.

If we unpack the word "Sên," we find it has many meanings, all of which are palpable and physical. Gross Sên are all things in the body that are stringy and noodle-like: a ligament, a nerve, a tendon, a vein, a capillary, a sinew, a strand of hair. Sên also describes the line of the horizon, a rope, wire, column, string, or thread. It does not describe **chi**, energy, vibration, or frequency. The *Royal Thai Dictionary* also describes Sên as being a measurement and "anything that has length without thickness": that is, it is a classifier (courtesy of Josh Jayindo, social media communication).

Side note: From a traditional medicine perspective, Fire and Wind elements can be classified as energy, as they are heat and movement; because of this, they are the functional and energetic aspects of the body.

Side note: The word "Sên" actually means pathway or, less accurately, "line." It is common to hear some practitioners say "Sên line" and not realize they are saying "line line." The most accurate translation from the Thai word to English is "pathway." In Thai medical texts, the word "**Naharu**" describes Sên being distorted and refers to actual physical structures in the body: for instance, damaged nerves or veins, or broken capillaries in the skin.

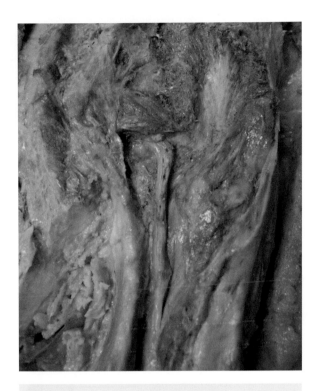

Fig. 10.2
The channels between the big muscles known collectively as the hamstrings. With kind permission of Functional Fascia.

Some gross Sên are very easy to locate and palpate, such as the Achilles tendon (calcaneal tendon) or the sciatic nerve. Sên can be treated directly with release points or with techniques such as plucking (see later). The techniques that address the Sên directly are often more uncomfortable than general channel work, as they focus on repositioning them and releasing them from the surrounding soft tissue.

In general channel work, a practitioner works by thumb pressing (see Chapter 20) on the myofascial connections between tissue and bone (for example, the tibialis anterior and the shin bone) or between two muscles (such as the biceps femoris and the semimembranosus

of the hamstrings; Fig. 10.2). These are areas where the practitioner can sink deeper into the body and where the underlying physical structures, known collectively as Sên, can be accessed as pathways of movement.

Muscle and Fascia

Muscle and fascia are both listed in the twenty body parts associated with Earth element (see Chapter 3). It is fascia that attaches muscle to bone and it can be found between all the major structures in the body. Tendons and ligaments are Sên, and both are fascia (Fig. 10.3).

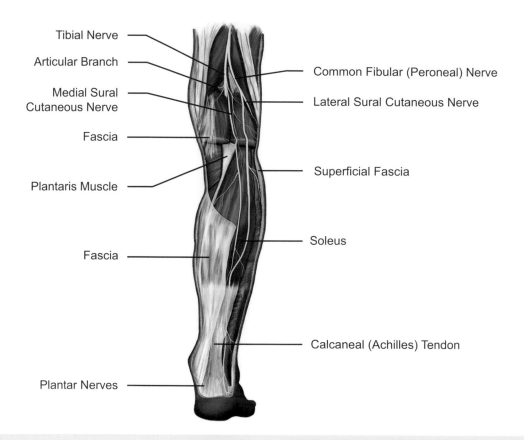

Tibial Nerve

Articular Branch

Medial Sural
Cutaneous Nerve

Fascia

Plantaris Muscle

Fascia

Plantar Nerves

Common Fibular (Peroneal) Nerve

Lateral Sural Cutaneous Nerve

Superficial Fascia

Soleus

Calcaneal (Achilles) Tendon

Fig. 10.3
Tendons and nerves on the posterior lower leg.

If you look at an anatomy book, you can see that skeletal muscles are striated. They wrap around the body in a spiraling pattern; there are no straight lines in the body. Each muscle is separated into its own container by epimysium, creating tiny fascia-filled spaces between them. Fascia is continuous throughout the body; like muscle tissue, it also wraps around, covers, and spirals in the body, encasing the muscles and supporting them. Muscle and fascia are intimately related everywhere in

the body; like everything in the internal landscape, they are co-dependent.

A useful way of picturing fascia and muscles is to peel an orange. To see what is inside we first have to take off the skin, just as you would have to do to look inside the body. What you will see in front of you is the fibrous layer, often a yellowy-cream color, that covers the fruit. This layer is similar to the superficial fascia that is tightly adhered to the skin. If you peel off this layer and open up the orange, you will see that the fruit is made up of segments, each of which is surrounded by a thin membranous layer. If you were to take one piece and open it, you would see that there are lots of tiny sacs, each covered in its own thin membrane. Muscles are just like this: they each have their own segment, and each striation also has a wafer-thin coating of fascia. Fascia and membranes both provide space between two things, isolating them from each other, often bone from tissue, or tissue from tissue.

Channels

Channels, **grooves**, valleys, or trenches are all useful nouns to describe the spaces in the body, but for ease and consistency I will call them channels. They are anatomical *physical* structures, not meridians or invisible pathways for energy. These channels are *gateways* to the Sên.

They are places on the body where hands often naturally migrate to when we are in pain, and want to press and knead.

During Thai bodywork, the practitioner focuses on the main channels but there are many more. Once one understands what a channel is, one can see and feel many of them in the body, all of which are on the edge of tendons, ligaments, muscles, or bone.

When the muscle or fascia feels bound up, tense, immobile, and unyielding, manual therapy helps to soften the tissue and make it more malleable. One of the main goals of Thai bodywork is to soften the muscle tissue and make more space in the fascia that separates the adjacent muscles, making sure there is no obstruction, so that Wind can move through the pathways.

Side note: Use your own body to explore these areas. Sit on the floor and bend your leg, keeping your foot on the floor, then place your hands on your hamstrings at the back of your upper leg; you will easily find these channels. Notice if different points along them feel hard, sore, and impenetrable, or maybe you observe that they are soft and malleable, or perhaps numb to sensation. Can you find four spaces between the big muscles there? Is there obvious isolated space between each of them? Are they easier to locate nearer to the knee or the sitting bones, or somewhere in the middle of the leg?

If muscles or fascia are hydrated and responsive, they have a yielding texture that is easily softened and that allows any touch to penetrate deeper into the body. If they are hard and bound up, there is naturally going to be less flow of blood and lymph or movement in them, and they will feel stiffer to the touch and palpation.

When a healthy, mobile body is touched, the channels can feel soft and malleable, with accessible spaces that the practitioner can sink into to penetrate deeper into the body. But if the fascia and soft tissue are bound up, the fibers become stuck and underlying structures, such as nerves and vessels, are also caught up in the harder tissue, resulting in them being less able to move freely and function optimally. This means that the practitioner will need to spend a lot of time addressing the muscle and fascia (second layer) to make more space in the channels for the Sên to have optimum function.

I like to use the analogy of a busy train, where you find yourself standing squashed between people who are so close that you can hardly move. This is how I imagine the Sên, surrounded by bound-up and unyielding muscle. When everyone gets off at the central station and the carriage empties out, you feel relief that you can move again and relax. When muscles are relaxed, the Sên have the freedom to function properly, something they cannot do when the muscle constricts them.

When your hands find areas that are stuck, solid, immobile, or stagnated, there can be many possible causes. There may be adhesions, injuries, scar tissue, or simply areas that have not had sufficient physical movement.

Another cause could be the subtle Winds (thoughts and emotions) which become physical (the thought that becomes a knot of tension, the fear that becomes an upset stomach, excitement that becomes butterflies). Daily habits and poor nutrients and nourishment also result in a build-up of toxins and a body that has excited or weakened Wind element. Persistent poor nutrition, unhealthy lifestyle, and lack of creative expression or self-care are all also causes of poor body function, lack of mobility, and a stiffening of the soft tissues.

The Thai physical therapist stimulates and treats Sên via the channels to stimulate or calm the movement of Wind element. In working at this level of physiology, with the intention of reaching the pathways of movement, the massage has a deep-rooted efficacy, delivering movement and touch input to the cells and organs of the physical body. Nerve impulses fire up, blood and nutrients can move through the body, lymph is cleared, toxins move.

Sên and Wind

Wind and movement are one and the same thing. The Thai word for Wind is "**Lom,**" and so Wind, Lom, and movement are all interchangeable terms.

Sên and **Wind** communicate throughout the whole body via the brain, central nervous system, and enteric system. Sên are also arteries, veins, and capillaries, part of the cardiovascular system and carriers of blood, nutrients, carbon dioxide, oxygen, and so on. Tendons and ligaments are also Sên; they have tensile strength (the movement of which is a type of Wind) while also allowing for movement.

All movement that happens in the body is Wind element, whether this takes the form of fingers typing on a keyboard, an unfertilized egg moving down through the fallopian tube, the movement of a thought that becomes an action, or the rhythm of the heartbeat. Sên are pathways for physical movements to happen. Wind is what brings the body to life.

When there is a depletion of movement in the Sên, weakened Wind element causes stagnation, pain, or dysfunction. An example of agitated Wind element causing imbalances would be restlessness, a heart that beats too fast (**tachycardia**), dizziness, erratic behavior, or too much movement in the body.

An interaction happening on a cellular level, a chemical exchange, a thought process, hormonal fluctuations, enzymes breaking down food, and an emotion are all examples of the subtle and invisible Wind moving through the body.

Arteries, nerves, lymph vessels, and tendons are the most gross and palpable Sên in the body, with big actions and movements. There are smaller branches of Sên, such as tiny nerves, vessels, capillaries, and neural off-shoots; these are still palpable and physical but on a more minuscule level.

There are also invisible movements taking place unconsciously in the body, such as changes in chemistry, hormones, digestive enzymes, and so on. The movement of a thought or emotion is also classified as Sên, although as a more subtle pathway, a movement of the mind.

The tangible, physical structure of all Sên is Earth element and is listed as an Earth body part. Any movement through Sên is Wind element. Each nerve, vessel, or capillary, no matter how small, has its own protective layer around it called the **endomysium**, which gives it elastic potential. It is like an electrical wire that has a rubber coating (fascia), but inside the tiny wire (Sên) it can transmit an electrical impulse and deliver communication (movement along the wire/Sên is Lom/Wind).

The invisible and subtle Sên are substances and processes that move through the gross Sên.

In Thai bodywork, healing the free flow of Wind is vitally important for the healthy function of the body on all levels. Like all the elements, Wind can be in various states, such as weakened, agitated, amplified, excited, distorted, or deranged. Bodywork techniques vary immensely with all the elements, depending on what is presenting, but especially with Wind element (see more on this in Chapter 4).

We need to be able to move easily and to express ourselves. Blood needs to flow to carry vital nutrients, nerves need to carry signals, food needs to be digested. If the Sên are clear, the body can be much more efficient.

It is often said that there are 72,000 Sên in the body; this is not really meant as a precise number, but more to give an idea of a countless number or immeasurable quantity. Picture in your mind the nerve or heart trees (see Fig. 10.1), the vast global connectors of movement that run throughout our human form. Add to this all the thousands of thought processes, hormonal fluctuations, chemical interactions, cellular activity, all the subtle and invisible movements of substances that are happening in any given moment in the body, and the significance and magnitude of Sên are easy to understand.

Working the Channels

Channel work takes focus, concentration, and practice, as the skill lies in its precision. There are many aspects to it and at first it may feel like awkward or hard work, but it is *so* worth putting in the time to ensure that it is accurate. This area of Thai bodywork effects physiological change, and the physiological response feels amazing to the recipient when it is carried out with skill. As we have noted, it sets Wind moving, connects the recipient to deeper aspects of themselves by waking up the body at a profound level, and frees it up in many therapeutic ways.

Chapter 10

Channels on the arms and legs can be worked in any position: side, prone, seated, or supine. In this book I will take you through the prone and supine position channel work of the lower limbs and arms.

To recap: the aim is to create space between structures, so when working next to a bone the angle will be away from bone, not on to it, as this would be closing not creating space.

One of the most important considerations is the direction of pressure into the channels, as this affects the accuracy of working on them and the feel of it for the recipient. Other considerations include how much to lean in to provide pressure; this is where being sensitive with your body, and confidence and practice come in. The more people you practice on, the more aware you become and the easier it is to know where the "bite" is. (I use the word "bite" but "end-feel" and "limit" are also accurate.)

Channel work is best learned directly from a teacher because of the high volume of fine details needed to make it accurate and effective. I have used muscles as a way to trace the channels, but it is important to remember that it is the spaces between the muscles that we are pressing on. Also, because muscles spiral and are layered, the channel often goes over or under the muscles I have mentioned.

There are many therapeutic ways to work the Sên and channels that do not involve using thumbs, but these require the instruction of a teacher for them to be safe and effective.

Positioning of Thumbs

For efficacy and optimum body mechanics, there is an ideal distance by which the thumbs should move when working on the channels. However, what I often see is that, instead of using the measurement as a guide, students will move their thumbs a tiny amount each time, which then tires them.

A general rule of thumb (excuse the pun) is to slide thumbs the distance between two knuckles each time. So, if your thumbs are placed with the ends touching, this will be the distance between the first knuckle of each thumb. There is a traditional measurement called "Anguli," which is that of a finger joint, and this is used for making infusions and **decoctions**, as well as for gauging distance on the body. For example, the distance between one thumb joint and the next is called an Anguli; this is useful to know when thumbing channels or finding release points.

Side note: This word is derived from the name Angulimala (meaning garland of fingers). Angulimala was a man who became a symbol of spiritual transformation. He was initially a ruthless law breaker, who was sent by a teacher to find a thousand human fingers, and in his quest he killed many people. He was almost killed himself but luckily was helped by the Buddha, who had such a gift for teaching and kindness that he was able to put him on the right path. Angulimala eventually ended up as a devout Buddhist and monk of the Theravada Buddhist tradition.

There are channels all over the body and specific directions for working on them (Fig. 10.4). These are easy to remember, as long as you are always pressing them to create space, not close it.

Legs (Fig. 10.5)

Supine Position

Side note: The hand position for thumbing is to use the flat of the thumbs and fingers as counterpressure. Keep the hands high so that the palm of the hand is not connected (Fig. 10.6).

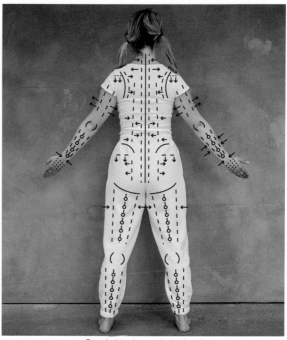

∘ Straight down into body
— Bone
-- Channel

Fig. 10.4
Channels and directions – the posterior body.

Inside lower leg

There are *two* main channels:

- *Location*: follow the line of the tibia, starting from below the medial malleolus (ankle bone). The tibia is wide and flat on the inside leg. To work this channel effectively, thumbs should stay close to the bone but not on it, and the pressure with thumbs is into the space between the bone and muscle.

75

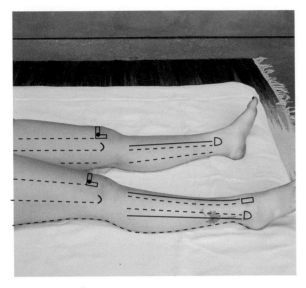

Bone ─────────── Bone
─ ─ ─ ─ ─ ─ ─ Channel

Squaring knee ⌐ Bony landmark – Inside upper
Outside upper

▭ Bony landmark – Outside lower

D Bony landmark – Inside and
outside lower

Fig. 10.5
Map of the leg channels.

- *Muscle*: soleus and gastrocnemius.

- *Angle*: the angle of pressure is rolling off the edge of the tibia. The thumbs should then press the tissue back up towards the bone into the small space.

- *Location*: the channel starts between the medial malleolus and Achilles tendon, then travels along the inside leg in the center of the belly of the muscle.

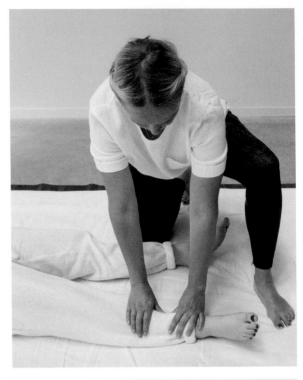

Fig. 10.6
Thumb work on the lower leg channels with high hands.

- *Muscle*: between soleus and gastrocnemius.

- *Angle*: straight into it, at 45 degrees.

Inside upper leg

There are *three* main channels:

- *Location*: square off the patella using your fingers. The starting point for your channel work is the precise right angle of the kneecap. This channel follows the edge of the femur.

- *Muscle*: vastus medialis.

- *Angle*: lean straight down on to it (Fig. 10.7).

- *Location*: find the soft dip between the patella, vastus medialis, and sartorius at the medial aspect of the knee.

- *Muscle*: sartorius/adductor longus/gracilis.

- *Angle*: down and away from the patella.

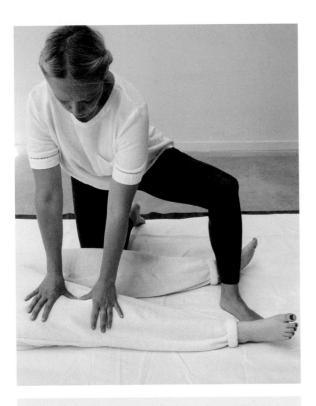

Fig. 10.7
Upper leg channel work with thumbs.

- *Location*: place the leg into a four position so the recipient's foot is close to their straight leg.

- *Muscle*: between semimembranosus and gracilis.

- *Angle*: 45 degrees, making sure you are not leaning weight down on to the leg but are pushing the leg away, abducting it. The recipient's knee will angle toward their head, opening up the hip joint as the thumbs press into the channel.

Outside lower leg

There are *three* main channels:

- *Location*: from the talocrural joint of the ankle bone, following the sharp edge of the tibia.

- *Muscle*: between tibia and fibula, tibialis anterior.

- *Angle*: straight down on to it.

- *Location*: find the upper edge of the lateral malleolus.

- *Muscle*: between extensor digitorum longus and peroneus longus.

- *Angle*: straight into it at 45 degrees.

- *Location*: begins between the posterior surface of the lateral malleolus and Achilles tendon.

- *Muscle*: fibularis brevis and longus.

- *Angle*: this channel is worked blind, as its location is posterior to the leg. The best way to find it is to identify the dip below the malleolus and follow it from there. Fingers should be on top and thumbs below, with hands internally rotated a little. The thumbs press up into the leg while the fingers squeeze, applying counterpressure. Often, the practitioner's elbows rest on their own leg, bent, as the angle is low.

Outside upper leg

There are *three* main channels:

- *Location*: square off the knee with the forefingers, making a right angle around the patella. This channel runs from the kneecap to the head of the trochanter.

- *Muscle*: vastus lateralis and tensor fasciae latae.

- *Angle*: straight down on to it, at 45 degrees.

- *Location*: find the soft dip at the side of the knee, femoral condyle.

- *Muscle*: iliotibial band.

- *Angle*: straight down on to it, at 45 degrees.

- *Location*: this channel is posterior and starts behind the back of the knee.

- *Muscle*: biceps femoris.

- *Angle*: up into it, using all fingers from both hands. Press up into the body (let the weight of the recipient's leg be what you

press into). The practitioner might rest the elbows on their own thighs for a comfortable working position.

Prone Position

Lower leg

There is *one* main channel:

- *Location*: straight up the middle of the lower leg, from the Achilles tendon and between the gastrocnemius heads.

- *Muscle*: gastrocnemius/soleus.

- *Angle*: down on to it.

Upper leg

There are *three* main channels:

- *Location*: straight up from the back of the knee to the ischial tuberosity.

- *Muscle*: between bicep femoris and semitendinosus.

- *Angle*: straight down on to it.

- *Location*: straight up the back of the leg.

- *Muscle*: between biceps femoris and vastus lateralis.

- *Angle*: medial move, straight into it, at 45 degrees.

- *Location*: the medial edge of the muscle group known as the hamstrings, starting about three fingers' width up (superior) from the knee.

- *Muscle*: between semimembranosus and gracilis.

- *Angle*: medial move, straight into it, at 45 degrees.

Arms

Supine Position

The inside arm should be massaged out-stretched to 45 degrees, palm upwards. The practitioner sits close to the recipient's body, facing their head.

Inside lower arm

There are *three* main channels:

- *Location*: from the wrist to the elbow between ulna and radius (Fig. 10.8).

- *Muscle*: between flexor carpi radialis and brachioradialis in the belly of the muscle.

- *Angle*: straight down on to it.

- *Location*: from the wrist joint to the elbow. These channels are found on either side of the radius and ulna bones.

- *Muscle*: flexor digitorum, flexor pollicis longus.

- *Angle*: work both channels at the same time with thumb and fingers; squeeze medially away from the bony landmarks.

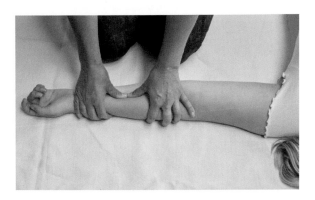

Fig. 10.8
The inside lower arm channel in the center of the forearm between ulna and radius.

Inside upper arm

There are *two* main channels:

- *Location*: starting under the pectoral muscles then continuing under the bicep to the elbow.

- *Muscle*: pectoralis major, biceps brachialis (Fig. 10.9).

- *Angle*: up and away from the bone.

- *Location*: below the humerus to the elbow.

- *Muscle*: triceps brachii.

- *Angle*: press away from bone.

Outside lower arm

The outside arm should be massaged beside the recipient's body, palm down. The practitioner sits next to their arm, facing it.

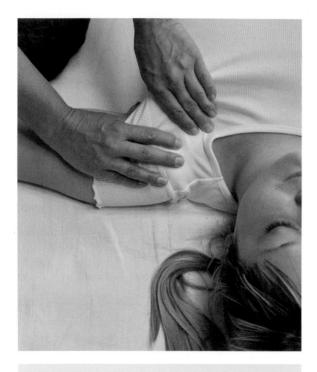

Fig. 10.9
The inside upper arm channel starts under the pectoral muscle and travels down under the biceps.

There are *three* main channels:

- *Location*: starting at the middle of the wrist joint and traveling up the center of the forearm.

- *Muscle*: between extensor digitorum and extensor carpi ulnaris

- *Angle*: down on to it.

- *Location*: from the wrist joint to the elbow. These channels are found on either side of the radius and ulna bones.

- *Muscle*: extensor carpi ulnaris, extensor carpi radialis brevis, extensor digitorum.

- *Angle*: work both channels at the same time with thumb and fingers; squeeze medially away from the bony landmarks.

Outside upper arm

There are *two* main channels:

- *Location*: following the line of the humerus from shoulder to elbow.

- *Muscle*: triceps brachii.

- *Angle*: into the channel and away from bone.

- *Location*: following the line of the humerus from shoulder to elbow.

- *Muscle*: biceps brachii.

- *Angle*: into the channel and away from bone.

Direct Sên Work

There are various techniques that can be used to work directly on the Sên. They are useful if a particular problem needs addressing directly, such as an impingement on a nerve or tendon that is restricting natural movement or causing pain.

One of my favorite Sên techniques is plucking. It can be painful, as it is performed with speed and repetition, but is very effective if carried out with skill. Often, when clients need it, they enjoy it, despite it being intense. You can find more information about this technique in Chapter 20.

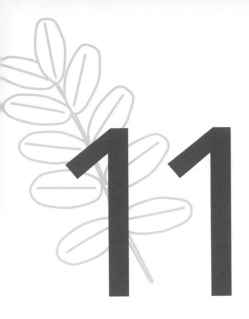

11

The Causes of Imbalance

The parallels between planet Earth and the body, and how they can both become out of balance, is striking. Just as in the natural world, all elements in the body simply exist. But as they fluctuate between various states of imbalance, they cause problems.

In an ideal world, we would experience balance and harmony between the four elements, and this is when we feel at our best. But, of course, this cannot be sustained throughout our whole lives. It is natural that, at times when an element becomes unbalanced, we experience suffering, weakness, vulnerability, agitation, or pain, and this can affect us mentally, emotionally, physically, and spiritually. When this happens, the body needs help to heal and repair itself, in much the same way that planet Earth does. The body and planet mirror each other with their various states of imbalance.

In Thai medicine, disease is seen as being caused by any of the forty-two elements of the body (twenty Earth element components, twelve Water element components, four Fire element components, six Wind element components).

A number of contributing factors cause imbalance and recognizing these helps when making a diagnosis for treatment. Here is an explanation of some of the causes.

Natural Elements and Their Balance

Many components influence our state of health, such as diet, sleep patterns, exercise, exposure to toxins, poor work environment, environmental temperature, and changes in weather. Natural urges, emotions, creative outlet, and posture also impact on us. The natural cycles of day and night, season, and age all affect our health. In Thai medicine, these are referred to as "natural causes." Influences of the Sun, Moon, and other planets in the solar system are also included in this.

A secondary cause of imbalance is seen as "unnatural." Ghosts or ancestral spirits, accidents, harm by weapons, and poisoning all fall into this category. Poisoning can affect any element in the body: think of cream that is applied to skin and causes a reaction, or rancid food that creates vomiting and diarrhea. Accidents and injury affect Earth element first – a broken bone, a cut to the skin, an inhaled substance that damages the lungs. Spirits and ghosts are powerful in that they can affect all elements, but as they are not tangible, they are most likely to affect the lightest element – Wind.

Karma is the tertiary cause of elemental imbalance. Past-life karma is said to influence our genetic make-up, so as we take our first breath we bring karmic history with us. Furthermore, our present-day actions, and how we choose to react and respond to the world we inhabit, have a direct impact. Our previous life and our present one affect future patterns.

In Thailand, spirits, deities, and ghosts can all cause disruption. Traditionally, there are specific bodywork practices and incantations that deal with these spirits before other bodywork is performed or herbal/dietary suggestions are made. Tok Sên (performed with a mallet and peg while incantations are silently repeated; Fig. 11.1), Sak Yan (spiritual tattoos; Fig. 11.2), Chet, and **Haek** (where a leaf is brushed over the body while an incantation is also silently repeated or whispered) are some examples.

Time

Following a twenty-four-hour time cycle, there are specific hours of the day and night when each element is at its most dominant. The twenty-four-hour cycle is traditional and relates to the Thai time cycle of day and night, but is adapted depending on the amount of hours that constitute day and night in other countries.

In Thailand, the elements Water, Fire, and Wind each have two cycles in the

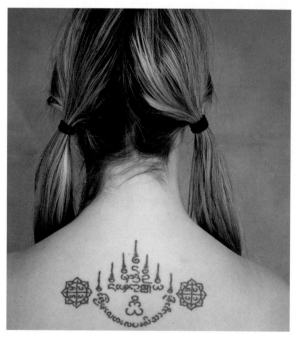

Fig. 11.2
Sak Yan spirit medicine tattoo uses medicinal herbs in the ink, Vedic astrology for the design, and incantations throughout the tattoo ritual.

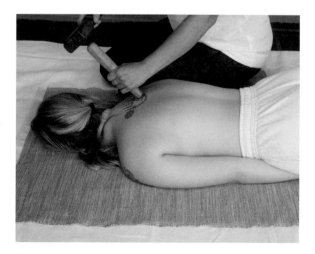

Fig. 11.1
Tok Sên tools are spirit medicine and also work on Sên with vibration.

twenty-four-hour period. This is useful to know when trying to ascertain which element is out of balance and causing a problem. The time of day when someone first noticed they were ill, or when a client feels at their best or worst, can help in diagnosis and gives valid insights as to why people may wake at a certain time in the early hours, or be hungry at a certain time in the afternoon, or feel more pain or tiredness. Alongside this, the time of day when someone was born, goes to bed, eats, exercises, wakes, and so on are all linked to time causative factors.

- Water   6–10 a.m. and 6–10 p.m.

- Fire   10 a.m.–2 p.m. and
               10 p.m.–2 a.m.

- Wind   2–6 a.m. and 2–6 p.m.

Season

The elements naturally fluctuate with the seasons, which can cause imbalances in our own body as it mirrors the natural world. Water element is more dominant in the colder months and reflects this element being a cold one. Fire is more noticeable in the hotter months, when the sun is stronger for longer. Wind dominates in the months where there is more rain (here we must think about the movement of the rain rather than the water itself). It is during the wetter season that we see more storms and strong winds.

Temperature

Exposure to heat or cold is a cause of imbalance. They are seen as pathogens to the body (and can be used to balance the body through bodywork tools and herbs).

Food

Eating food that is rotten or fermented, or eating blood or parts of animals seen as "improper," causes sickness and imbalance. Fermented foods, eating at certain times of day when digestion is slow, and over-eating are considered to be causes of imbalance related to the digestive Winds. This is also seen as a cause of pain in the joints and muscles of the body due to improper nutrients traveling through the body systemically.

Age

The elements are more dominant at certain times in our lives. Similar to how the moon waxes and wanes, one element slowly increases as another decreases. For example, little children tend to be at the Wateriest time of their lives. It is easy to see this: they tend to have big eyes and soft, fluid bodies, they cry a lot and are emotional, and they are malleable (think about how bendy their bodies are and how they are easily distracted). This is also a time when they are more prone to Watery conditions, where they have a lot of mucus, or are teething and dribbling.

Waxing and Waning

Children go through a stage where their Water element is decreasing but their Fire element is increasing, from their early teens into their early twenties. They still have many

Water-dominant characteristics, but as these decrease, Fire element is gaining momentum. It can be a difficult time while these natural fluctuations are occurring, as it brings such change, and these changes can be dramatic.

Teenagers have strong opinions. They are often frustrated, angry, passionate, and strong-willed, starting to really know their own minds and not afraid to show their feelings and speak out. It is also a time when hormones are increasing and changing, and becoming more dominant; there are skin changes and often an increase in rashes, spots, and oily skin. These are common characteristics of a Fiery time of life. There is a stronger focus on sexual awakening and awareness during this transformative period.

As teenagers turn into young adults, they become more stable in their Fire element, being driven, decisive, and action-based. As they move through their Fire-dominant years and Wind becomes more pronounced, it is common to see subtle changes in mind-set with Fire waning.

Later in life, Wind becomes more dominant. The skin becomes drier, and people suffer more with aches and pains or disrupted sleep. Sensitivities to foods or noise become much more frequent and commonplace.

These influences are important to acknowledge, as they help us form a clearer picture of the recipient's predispositions (core element constitution, CEC; see Chapter 5) and of the contributing factors that might be causing current imbalances, conditions, and suffering. Each of these factors and other more causative ones can be studied in further depth (see Resources for further reading).

Wind Element

In Thai medicine, more diseases are linked to the Winds than any other element. There are over 80 diseases attributed to the Winds and there are 108 Winds in the body. This number represents an infinite number, but if we were to count how many movements there are through the physical and subtle Winds, it might not be far off.

The gross Winds are attributed to the physical body. The subtle Winds are the movements of the mind; they are not physical and cannot be palpated. Meditation is the tool that can calm and balance the subtle Winds.

The Winds are also categorized more specifically into:

- *Course Winds* – these move primarily through the main channels of the digestive system.

- *Mild Winds* – these are the Winds that move through the blood vessels.

- *Fine Winds* – these are the neural impulses and communication pathways moving through the nervous system.

- *Sense Winds* – these correspond to the sense organs.

- *Karmic Winds* – these define the time of death, lifetime patterns, and rebirth.

There are three primary disease-causing Winds that are responsible for imbalance and which are collectively called Vāyo. These are different to Wind related to the element. **Vāta** is the Pali word for Wind.

- *Heart Wind* – this Wind circulates around the body. It is the Wind of the heart and breath. The Heart Wind distributes the essence of the heart and has the role of protecting it.

- *Knife-like Wind* – this Wind is related to pain in the digestive system and is responsible for overall pain in the body.

- *Central Channel Wind (Sumana)* – this relates to the gross movement of Wind throughout the central channel of the body (posterior and anterior: that is, the spine and aorta, and all other Sên in this area. Remember that this is a highly innervated and vascular area of the body).

Wind Disease

Wind disease arises in the first four layers of the body and from the blood and heart.

The blood is often cause of disease – it is an extraordinary fluid in the body, as it has three elements attributed to it.

The heart (which is connected strongly to the mind) is the primary organ where Wind disease starts to ascend from.

Toxic Winds

These are the winds that cause trembling, diarrhea, fever, and vomiting.

12

Love Your Guts

Did you know that much of your belly is in your back? Not many people realize that the intestines, even in a small person, would span the length of a car if laid out in a line. This helps give a sense of their dimensions and of how cleverly they are tucked neatly away with the other organs, filling the large, cavernous space between diaphragm and pelvic bowl.

Some of the tissues in the belly, such as the superficial fascia which is attached and deep to the skin, should be lubricated and slippery, able to slide and move. There is a membranous layer called perifascia which allows for the differential movement, so that when we stretch and move, these layers can glide.

Some backache can be caused by deeper tissues in the belly, like the intestines being stuck together and not moving. Just as in any other area, things can get bound up and adhesions can form.

Another reason why it is important for your innards to be correctly in situ, soft, and malleable is so that ingested food can slide on through from mouth to anus (making its way down the gastro-intestinal tract), and nutrients can be extracted along the way. Just as in any other area in the body, if there are restrictions, the pathway is not going to function at its peak.

Side note: Food moves through the gastro-intestinal tract by wave-like concentric contractions called "peristalsis." (The message for movement comes from a neural impulse (Sên), the movement of the muscle is Wind element, and the smooth muscle is Earth element.)

The intestines are organized in such a way that they can resemble an abundant bunch of flowers. In a dissection, it is possible for your hands to reach to the root of the mesentery and lift it up in its entirety, like a bouquet. The first time I did this, it was the most surprising vision, reminding me of a magician pulling flowers from a hat, and it was as delightful. The unraveling continues long after it seems possible. Once the intestines are removed, the weight of them is astonishing. It often takes more than one pair of hands to hold them for any length of time.

The intestines are also very beautiful. At first, when full, they may resemble sausages, but they can be opened and cleaned up, and in doing so, the **villi** are exposed. To the eye, these are very similar to underwater coral, with an "imperfectly perfect" continuous pattern like trees laid down flat on a forest floor. The villi do the job of pushing things through.

The tubular-shaped intestines are attached at the root by the mesentery. This is a membrane that is rich in vasculature and in endocrine and immune cells, and has lymph nodes in it; it draws nutrition from the intestinal wall to the body. It has an unusual texture, as it looks fatty but has more substance than superficial fascia. There are fairly thick vessels intrinsically embedded within, and when held up and back-lit it is beautiful, like an arcade of vasculature or a scallop shell. In the dissection lab I have heard it called "brain coral" by Gil Hedley, who acknowledges its integral intelligence.

There are many more structures in the belly and it is worth exploring them from superficial to deep because it is exactly how you will treat the area. As with any area of the body, we start at the skin and work our way deeper.

Here I would like to note that Thai anatomy does not class structures in the same way that a Western anatomist would. To work with the body, we must observe and palpate, and let go of trying to understand the body through the minutiae, or to make the Western anatomy fit with the Thai viewpoint.

In a cadaver lab, the layers are sometimes dissected with the hands, which can be used like a blunt instrument, or with other sharper or heavier tools like a scalpel or cutters, for example. It is very much dependent on what the enquirer is reflecting, and the sculpture they are making and exposing. Layers are textural and energetically diverse; they vary in quality. But really, there is not one separate part, component, or process in the body from subtle to gross, from superficial to deep, from conceptual to matter.

Skin – First Layer

The skin is our body's natural wetsuit. It is one continuous layer, with no gaps, parts, or breaks. It is waterproof, which ensures that gases or liquids are not able to penetrate the surface of the body. However, there are specific cells within the skin that are absorbent and produce lipids. These cells go straight to the bloodstream (hence the skin can be used to make therapeutic herbs penetrate the body).

The skin of the arm is the same skin as that of the belly. Yet there are different **accessory cells** in specific areas, such as under the armpits where sweat glands produce sweat.

The skin is one huge beautiful organ, rich in neural offshoots and capillaries. When dissected and held up to the light, it is subtly patterned and light can shine through it. Take a moment to appreciate that when the sun shines, we are being illuminated inside as we absorb the vitamins from the rays of the sun.

Soft Tissue, Muscle, Fascia – Second Layer

Superficial fascia is the layer directly deep to and continuous with the skin. It is yellow in color and sponge-like in texture, having an oily and slippery feel. This layer is often the one that gives someone their shape. It varies in thickness and is like a fleecy or spongy body-suit on the well-nourished person, but can be a "sliver" of a layer on a thin body – so thin that it is almost impossible to separate from the skin in a dissection.

The superficial fascia is often called the "fat layer," which does not have much of an appreciative ring to it. The word "fat" does not accurately describe the superficial fascia, which is an astonishing endocrine gland and also a protective layer full of lymph nodes.

Side note: The **peritoneum** is a smooth and transparent membrane of filmy fascia that facilitates movement of the superficial fascia over the deep fascia that encases the muscles. It is a **serous membrane** that is lubricated and is made of the same fabric as the pericardium and pleura.

Deeper still, we find the abdominal muscles. For many people, it is easy to conjure up an image of these, both from anatomy books and from the pictures of well-defined bellies that are prevalent in the media everywhere we look. The first time I saw these muscles I was amazed at how uninteresting and unimpressive they appeared: thin and meaty, with striations that reminded me of food that has had a fork run through it to create a stripy pattern. These units of muscle are called **sarcomeres** and are represented by stripes of muscle with enclosing fascia, between each one and at each end of it, keeping them connected but separate, organized, and layered.

Side note: There are deeper abdominal muscles, such as the transversus abdominis, which wrap around the torso and have horizontal striations. Deep to the viscera there are muscles such as the psoas and quadratus lumborum, which cannot be directly touched as they are so deep. However, the fascia that surrounds the psoas is in direct continuity with that of the viscera and the **crus** of the diaphragm (see Chapter 8).

The membranous sac is a fairly thin membranous and continuous layer called the peritoneum. It is found lining the abdominal wall, not only at the front of the body (parietal peritoneum/sac) but at the back, too, where it is called the retro-peritoneum. It continues as the visceral peritoneum between and encasing organs, holding them in place like little supporting envelopes. The organs are closely and densely packed and organized. They do not become stuck, as they have a thin layer of peritoneal fluid around them.

To my knowledge, the sac is not mentioned specifically in Thai medical theory but would be seen as part of the second layer, as it is soft tissue/fascia.

When we open up the sac, we can see the **greater omentum** (Fig. 12.1). This has often migrated to an organ and wrapped itself around it, and because of this it can be elusive and not always easy to spot immediately. It can be tucked away and folded over on itself down into the pelvis, or it can be flat and up by the diaphragm, or anywhere in between.

Chapter 12

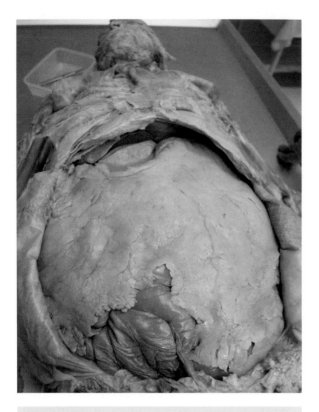

Fig. 12.1
The greater omentum. By special permission of Functional Fascia.

Every time I have been in the dissection lab, I have been fascinated by the greater omentum, so much so that I have now studied quite a few. Not one of them has ever looked the same as the next. The shape and size of the omentum vary from one person to another: sometimes thick, fatty, and sponge-like, at other times like a wafer-thin, fatty sheet. The variations in shape, girth, color, texture, and location are a constant surprise and one that reminds me to remain both interested and humble. In the living, it is completely mobile, but when there is a problem such as a burst appendix or perforation it will move to help the inflammatory response. The omentum, when passive and not needed in its healing role, will move passively because of the intestine (that is deep to it) moving beneath it.

The greater omentum is an amazing bit of internal architecture, in its design and function. If you ever needed convincing that there was reason to appreciate your belly, this is it. Here's why …

The greater omentum is a quadruple layered fold of peritoneum (connective tissue) and is a wonderful fatty and vascular structure that can migrate and move, lengthen and fold itself up. This part of the mesentery drapes down in the abdominal cavity like an old-fashioned apron. It lies under the muscles and covers the viscera. It has the ability to detect an organ that needs help and then moves to it and covers it over, wrapping it up like a comfort blanket. To describe its function in very simple terms: it absorbs waste, reduces inflammation, and promotes healing.

"[The greater omentum is] a wonderful moving fleece comforting the downtrodden of the abdominal visceral space like a mendicant Doctor, moving towards and wrapping organs in distress, reducing inflammation, and functioning like a clay poultice drawing out toxins as a lymphoid organ. It is comprised of prolongations of the visceral peritoneum of the stomach and the transverse colon, draping from these like a warm blanket over the intestines. Love your greater omentum, it serves you in your greatest need!"

Gil Hedley, personal communication, 2020

The greater omentum has been used very successfully after spinal surgery, an ingenious surgeon thinking outside the box and using its anti-inflammatory function to speed up his patient's recovery time, wrapping it around the area to heal it. More often, it is used in gastro-intestinal surgery to protect and heal: for example, after a perforation has been stitched or after a section of the bowel has been resected.

By the time we reach this layer in the lab, navigating inner space, it is easy to lose ourselves in the excitement that this deep visceral layer brings. There is a tangibly different "vibe" in the lab as this area is explored and appreciated. I notice a similar feeling in the room when students learn to give visceral massage. There is a deepening of respect for the body as they work on the vital organs and the layers from superficial to deep.

Sên and Channels – Third Layer

In Thai medicine, the Sên are taught as being arranged around the navel like a wheel. From what I have seen in the lab, there is, in fact, a vast amount of nerves and vessels in this area (neuro-vascular bundles/Sên), which makes it a significant area for communication to the whole body and for movement of Wind through the pathways. The superficial myofascial channels are located at the edge of the muscles (rectus abdominis, transversus abdominis, and straight down the middle at the **linea alba**, a flat, tendinous, fascial midline on the abdominal wall that runs from the xyphoid process to the pubic symphysis). There are deeper Sên activated by working on the **pulses**. The channels originate at the navel in embryonic development.

The gastro-intestinal system has its own nervous system called the enteric nervous system (ENS). This functions autonomously and yet also communicates with, and is influenced by, the central nervous system (the brain and spinal cord). The neurons and plexuses of the ENS are embedded in the walls of the gastro-intestinal tract from esophagus to anus. Within the walls of these organs is a unique and complex network of neurons (Sên). This area is often called the "first, second or gut brain" (depending on who is doing the talking).

In Thai medical terminology, this area is defined as being rich in gross and subtle Sên, it being highly innervated and full of arteries and veins. The cardiovascular and neural trees feed, clean, move, and nourish vital blood and messages around the body in an amazing network from superficial to deep.

The ENS is part of the autonomic nervous system, which is also made up of the sympathetic and parasympathetic nervous systems. Between them, they control breathing, heart rate, and response to stress, and initiate repair. The ENS has constant two-way communication with the central nervous system, yet is highly unusual as it can also function independently of it. This is a highly intelligent and intuitive part of the body and is also is a chemical and hormonal messenger. The ENS is so rich in neurons that it has more than the spinal cord: somewhere in the region of 100 million.

There is a general increasing fascination with the clear messages that the gut gives and how the brain and gut interact. Cast your mind back to a time when you were stressed out. No doubt one of the first ways you took notice of a physical response to this stress would have been an upset, tense, or nauseous tummy. Think how many times you have been nervous and then felt nauseous, or felt those butterflies that flutter when you are excited or on edge. This clearly shows the psychosocial influence on the actual physiology of the gut.

Decisions are often made on "gut feeling," yet the brain and the gut are working in synchronicity. Both are dealing with incoming sensory information from present and previous experience. This connection between the ENS and the brain is not metaphorical. The intrinsic and consistent information travels along the Sên (pathways of movement), which form a vast network in the body.

Gross Sên

As we have seen, the abdomen is home to a vast amount of Sên (there is often mention of 72,000 Sên in the body). This area is so rich in nerves and vessels that it would be accurate to say a huge percentage of Sên lie in this area, from superficial to deep, all of which originated in the navel in embryonic development.

Because of this, it is an area that can be worked on to access and treat the gross and subtle Sên. In Thai medicine, the source of all problems meets the channels in the gut (Fig. 12.2).

Abdominal Aorta

This is the main artery that feeds the abdominal organs. It is located deep to the small intestines and lies anterior to the vertebrae. There is a strong pulse located at the navel. This physical structure of this artery is called **Sên Sumana** in Thai medicine.

Whatever the CEC of your client, whatever their state of health or imbalance, working on the belly will bring balance and calm, nourishment and space to this area. (See Chapter 22 for more information.)

Elements and the Gut

The element associated with the *structure* of these internal organs, the surrounding fascia and muscle, is Earth. Interestingly, the **chyme** is also considered an Earth body part, as once food has been ingested, it becomes part of the body. The waste product of this element is feces.

The fluids, such as the lubricating oils, bile, mucus, and saliva, are all Water element. The abdomen is seen as an area where Water element is concentrated.

The impetus and digestive fire needed to break down food are Fire element. The organs where Fire is most concentrated are the liver (called hard liver in Thai medicine), gall bladder, and small intestines (consider the heat of

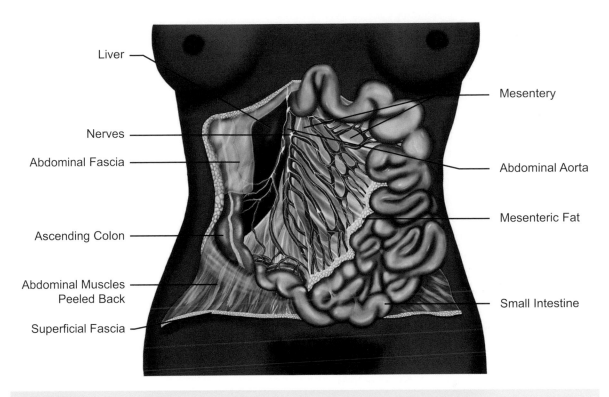

Fig. 12.2
The internal architecture of the abdomen.

Labels: Liver, Nerves, Abdominal Fascia, Ascending Colon, Abdominal Muscles Peeled Back, Superficial Fascia, Mesentery, Abdominal Aorta, Mesenteric Fat, Small Intestine

bile production that helps to break down food). And specifically, there are the adrenal glands and the pancreas (called soft liver in Thai medicine), organs that deal with absorption and chemical and hormonal response. The kidneys sit on the posterior abdominal wall against the back muscles, on either side of the spine in the upper abdominal area. They have a fatty subserosal fascia that packs around them. The adrenals are nestled inside the upper portion of the kidneys. When someone is stressed, the adrenals pump out epinephrine (adrenaline) as part of the fight or flight response of the sympathetic nervous system, making us ready for action. This could explain why there is often an element of power or Fire associated with this area of the body, and why it can be cultivated as an internal source of energy.

Peristalsis and the movement of food through the digestive tract is Wind element (remember that all movement is Wind). Fire element is primarily responsible for the breakdown of food. The food itself is Earth element. The digestive juices and the ability for the food to slide through the digestive system are Water element.

Side note: If we think about food (in its natural state), we can see it as medicine for our body. When we eat plants (Earth element from the ground) or meat (the Earth element of animals), they become part of us and can help heal Earth element in us.

Side note: Someone who is apple-shaped is likely to be presenting their viscera to the world. It is normal and healthy for there to be a measure of fat within the abdominal space and for it to present itself differently (individually, elementally, and constitutionally).

"People can be overweight in many ways: in the greater omentum, around the kidneys, etc. In all of the places where it is good and normal for adipose to be present, it can also be present in over-abundance. That being said, what is a healthy amount is very specific to the individual, and can vary greatly. Health expresses itself in many different body shapes and sizes."

Gil Hedley, personal communication, 2018

Side note: In Thai medicine, the abdomen has been seen for thousands of years as a great source of channels, and as the area of the mother pulse. Other pulses go to the legs, arms, and head, which is why there is a five-limb pulse diagnosis in Thai traditional medicine.

General Contraindications to Visceral Treatment

- Swelling of organs.

- Pregnancy.

- Inflammation.

- Kidney stones.

Side note: There are some other cautions and contraindications for visceral treatment and I recommend professional training before undertaking this work in clinic.

13

Disease Through the Layers

What happens when pathogens or disease enter the body? How can bodywork or medicinal herbs help?

In Thai medicine, pathogens or disease-causing factors are always condensing or dispersing. As they condense, they become deeper and slower, moving through the elements. As they densify, they become more physical and have the potential to be more serious.

One of the many goals of Thai bodywork is to draw pathogens from deep in the body and reverse the pattern of condensation, supporting and encouraging the body by dispersing those that were causing sickness and ill health. The body has an astonishing ability to heal, but sometimes it needs a helping hand to dissipate or break down what is causing it to be ill. In Thai medicine, heat, cold, toxins, lack of movement, dampness, and Wind are all classified as pathogens.

A thought can become a sensation in the body. Unless there is an injury, a physical pain comes from a thought. The thought is Wind element, the lightest of the four elements that make up the physical body. As the thought slows down, it becomes less energetic and turns into an emotion. Fire is the element of transformation, so as the thought slows further and meets Water element (also an element of emotion) it starts to be a physical experience in our gross anatomy, Water and Earth. This is why stress, being under pressure, or a fear of something can end up being a physical experience, felt in the body as a pain in the shoulders, a tension headache, or a cramp in the stomach. Although the pain itself is Wind element, the physicality of it is Earth element. The shoulders, head, and stomach are all more tense, and the Earth element body part is more solid and constricted. This is where bodywork or herbs can lend a helping hand. The practitioner can utilize various manual therapy tools or herbal medicine to help the body repair.

In bodywork, we break up and dissipate that which has become physical, such as adhesions, stagnation, areas where there is no movement, and places where fluids and blood are stuck. We help to draw out heat or dampness from the body by bringing these to the skin to help it perform its eliminatory function. We use heat to warm the body with compresses and medicinal heating balms.

Chapter 13

A Real-Life Example

I will use a real-life experience to give an idea of the potential progress of disease through the physical body from a Thai medicine perspective. In understanding this, it is possible to see how Thai bodywork can help reverse accumulation, disperse a build-up of toxins, and support the body in its healing process.

I was in the South of France on holiday, enjoying the sunshine and the heat. On this particular day, I had been lying in the sun for a few hours, engrossed in a book. I was not thinking about being out in the midday sun. I knew I was really hot, yet I ignored the warning signals and carried on reading, trying to reach the end of the chapter before lunch was called.

A little later, it was time to eat and I sat down with my family. The food was on the table when I suddenly felt *extremely* weak; all the energy had drained out of my muscles. I excused myself and managed to climb upstairs, shivering and feeling sick. For the next seven hours I lay on the bed, cold, nauseous, and aching in my muscles and joints. The overriding and most worrying feeling was that I was drifting out of my physical body. It was only when my young daughter kept reappearing at the door to check on me that I came back into my body. It took many days for the dizziness to disappear and in retrospect I can see that I felt weakened and depleted for some time after.

At the time, I had no idea of a progression of disease or the longer-term effects this experience would have on my body; nor did I know that my body would have benefited from a cooling internal herb such as **Andrographis**. This could have helped my body process the heat toxin. A scraping tool (Khuut) would also have been of assistance if I had used it to scrape my head and let some heat out.

For a couple of years after this, if there was any rise in temperature from the sun above about 20 degrees, I would start to sense danger. I found myself avoiding being exposed to it *at all* and realized I had become literally scared of the sun. My nervous system sensed danger; cellular memory suspected further threat.

Over the following months, I noticed that my hormones were affected with unusually erratic menstruation. My heart rate was often fast. In Thai medical terms, this indicates heat toxins in the body (remember that heat and cold can both be pathogens). Yet I often felt cold, as if my blood was not able to heat. The skin on my face rapidly changed, and I went from having a clear and smooth complexion to experiencing discoloration and pigmentation. Both the lack of heat in my body and the rapid transformation of my skin indicated distorted Fire element. I did not attribute this to the sunstroke, but in hindsight I can see that it was a possible cause.

What you can see from this experience is that the heat was a pathogen entering my skin, which traveled to my muscles, causing pain and weakness. It then progressed deeper to the Sên (nerves, vessels, and so on), where movement (Wind element) was impeded. The bone layer was affected, making my joints ache, and then the discomfort quickly progressed to the organ layer, the glands, brain, and heart.

How Thai Bodywork Can Help

In this somewhat extreme example, Thai bodywork could have been helpful. The eliminatory properties of skin could have been utilized if scraped or cupped, which would have drawn heat out of my body. Cooling internal herbs and water would have been the first port of call to support the reaction of heat in my body by calming Fire element. In theory, these could have helped my body to quickly deal with and disperse the pathogen (the heat) that was making me suffer.

Another example of how Thai bodywork can be used to dissipate is in the case of somebody getting soaked by the rain, resulting in catching a chill. The skin gets cold, and the cold permeates the underlying layer by making the muscles stiff and sore. This stiffening of the soft tissue would affect Wind element (when muscles are tight and cannot move easily, this is impeded Wind element, as the contraction of a muscle is movement). Ideally, this is the point at which a Thai bodyworker would be involved, massaging the tissue layer with heated herbal compresses, beating, kneading, and adding heating balms to encourage movement back into the muscle and fascia. This would free up the soft tissue and enable work to take place in the channels and Sên, restoring the healthy free flow of Wind through the deeper structures. If left untreated, the progression could continue to the Sên with blockages in vessels, blood, and lymph, or neural impingement. Bodywork could address this layer, initially with some mild massage and use of compresses and later, as the body begins to recover, with deep thumb compressions to the channels. Lack of movement is one of the ways that we are most likely to experience a build-up of stagnation (movement is the key to hydration and the flow of fluids in the body). The build-up tends to happen in weak areas and often accumulates where there are bends or naturally less blood flow, such as at the joints (bone layer). In massage, this layer is addressed and cared for by range of motion and traction techniques. If there is impeded Wind element, range of motion is especially helpful, as it inputs movement (Wind) into the body. If the cold went to the organ layer, the lungs might be affected (a cough). Fever is produced by the hypothalamus in the brain and is agitated Fire element.

The progression of disease, however, does not always start with the skin and it does not always affect the organs. If toxins are inhaled or ingested, they travel quickly to the organ layer, such as with food poisoning or smoking. Organs that have a connection to the external world are known as "open organs." These are the lungs (via the trachea) and stomach (via the esophagus), and they will be affected first. The solid organs that are "landlocked" are affected last.

In these cases, a practitioner would use herbs to nourish, support, and eliminate as necessary, alongside bodywork techniques such as cupping and scraping to draw out the pathogens.

In Thai bodywork, we need to think about how disease enters the body to cause harm, and how we as bodyworkers can focus on dissipating this. This could be with hands that create more movement in the tissue, but equally with fire cupping that draws pathogens from within the body.

14 Stretching and Movement

"Lazy person's yoga" – how I have come to loathe this phrase as a way to describe Thai bodywork.

I hear the expression used so frequently, making it appear that the yoga-like stretches are the only distinctive and noteworthy elements of the massage, totally without regard for the multiple tools a Thai healing arts practitioner might use. Another important point is that this phrase is actually inaccurate, as the recipient should be physically engaged in the "stretch" to some degree: that is, they might be holding the practitioner's arm or making an exhalation. They should always be participating with their own personal awareness of each stretch as it is applied because they are ultimately the authority on their own body and will know if they are being taken out of a comfortable range.

As a reader of this book, it is likely that the applied yoga stretches caught your eye and you were understandably impressed by their visual beauty. Or perhaps the idea of your body being stretched into a pretzel appeals, and you think it will feel good and have a huge therapeutic impact? Maybe you want to be able to bend, lift, and stretch a partner in all the delightful ways that one can if one knows how. This is something I come across all the time: it is the stretches that seem to catch people's interest. They are impressive, but are not what Thai massage is all about. Stretching is merely one tool: sometimes helpful but at other times not indicated at all.

Let's unpack this a little …

For many years, the treatments I gave to clients consisted of a high percentage of stretches that were part of a sequence. The one aspect of the sequence that varied each time was the stretching. I adapted the sequence as I saw fit for the individual, but also because the stretches sometimes had an impressive or **acroyoga** style appeal to them. The recipient would often be surprised by how their body could be stretched into many different positions.

But in retrospect I came to realize that these big, dynamic, and impressive stretches are *not often* very therapeutic, and despite being pleasurable to receive and fun to give, they were largely ineffectual. I started to recognize that, for my practice to grow and for my treatments to be effective, I needed to refine things and learn more about the body.

Nowadays, all of the complicated and impressive stretches I once used have been put away at the back of my toolbox, rarely surfacing in a treatment session unless necessary (or if I want to demonstrate what can be done, for fun). However, I still have great appreciation for the number of ways that two bodies can work together, and the shapes and movements that are made from this interaction (Fig. 14.1).

Generally, I use fewer stretches, most of which are fairly simple and concentrate on one muscle group (rather than targeting many muscle groups in one go). I stretch the people I see who *need* stretching, as not everybody does (see Chapter 4 for more on this).

The mind-set of "attaining flexibility" that has developed over the years can be

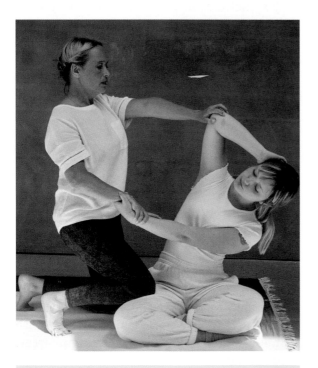

Fig. 14.1
Targeted stretch for the latissimus dorsi.

quite problematic. There is a current trend towards stretching longer and harder, but in truth this can be damaging and counterproductive. If one imagines hair curled into ringlets, it is possible to pull it and make it straight. When the tension is released, it springs back to its original shape or resting place. If you repeatedly pull the hair, it will eventually lose its potential to spring back as quickly, and while it may return some of the way, it will temporarily not recoil all the way back to its original state of tension or natural resting place. It has lost the ability to spring back, compromising its structural integrity. This results in less storage of energy, which weakens the muscle's reaction time and increases the risk of injury.

"If we become overstretched, over time we can lose that 'spring back' facility if tissues are repeatedly forced to exceed their elastic limit. Plastic deformation becomes irreversible … then damage can occur in the form of a tear, a break or snapping of a tendon."

Joanne Avison, 2015

I noticed this in my own body after two years of regular yoga. I constantly suffered from a vulnerable back and could not run in the park without my knees feeling pain and weakness. I realized that all the stretching of my naturally bendy body was making it lose strength around the joints. Once I noticed this, I suddenly became acutely aware that I was seriously loose to the point at which I felt had reduced the muscular and fascial support around the joints.

Is Bending Like a Pretzel a Good Thing?

I would answer with an outright "no." I am in favor of movement and a good range of motion: for example, being able to reach for things on a high shelf or bending easily to pick something off the floor. These might not be impressive, but they are functional and necessary movements that the body needs for daily life. I cannot see much use in being able to wrap the leg around the head. I think we need a balance of mobility and strength for optimal health in our tissues.

"If we were too 'elasticated' we could not function: the energy literally leaks."

Joanne Avison, 2015

Focused therapeutic stretching of the receiver's body creates space in the tissues and hydrates them through movement. This can activate many wonderful interoceptive feelings, which arise from the stretch sensations that ripple through the body. They happen when the soul is supported into a deepened, relaxed state and the dehydrated area of the body starts to feel itself being moved and touched, and becoming juicy again (Fig. 14.2).

What are Healthy Tissues?

Healthy range in the body is one that is balanced between flexibility and mobility, and that also incorporates stability and strength. The balance of fluid in the tissue is a contributing factor for function at an optimum level. Temperature, hydration, movement, electrolytes,

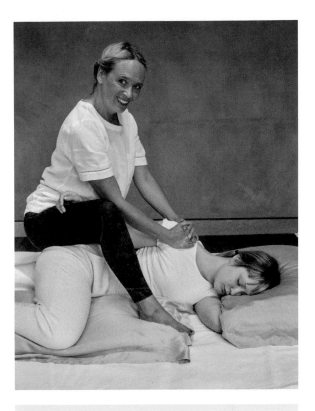

Fig. 14.2
Targeted stretch for the trapezius.

nutrition, creativity, love, self-expression, and happiness – these all affect the health of the whole body.

The **Piezo electric** Effect is an electrical charge that resides within bone and fascia, storing energy. Prolonged stretching could easily damage and weaken this integral system as the tensile properties of the tissues alter. When moving, healthy tissues naturally press and squeeze, slide and glide, which generates an electrical current. In this optimal environment, soft tissues have an easy, fluid, and hydrated quality to them. When

Chapter 14

manual therapy is applied to the tissues and they become more pliable, there is a knock-on effect on all other pathways of movement and a healthier (Piezo electric) charge is generated.

The tissues in the body that are mainly affected by "stretching" or "elongating" are fascia and connective tissue (and the nervous system also responds to and controls this movement). It is fascia that surrounds, supports, and interweaves its way through muscle, giving it both strength and movability. When we think of stiff, tight muscles, we are actually feeling our fascial fabric being tightly wound. If these tissues cannot contract fully, they also cannot relax sufficiently to a neutral position. Without movement, these tissues will become dehydrated, and then there is a catch-22 situation whereby they can neither expand or contract, so any movement becomes painful; they then move even less, causing more pain, and so on. This is one of the areas where Thai massage shines. It has the ability to rehabilitate movement and retrain the nervous system to allow for extra range, albeit passively – at least to begin with. In fact, there is a good reason why passive movement is so effective.

What is Happening During Passive Stretching?

One of the benefits of Thai massage stretches is that they are done passively; there is almost no active motor engagement (it is only under anesthesia that there is no motor engagement or muscle tone at all). The receiver's body is in a relaxed state and is not using muscle

strength or control for any of the movements. The experience of being passively stretched is very different to stretching oneself, as the muscles and surrounding fascia can relax and be in a resting state. The relaxed tissues can easily be taken to contraction and lengthening, and then returned again to a relaxed, neutral point through a passive stretch.

Muscles do not lengthen dramatically through stretching. While it might feel fantastic, their structure does not change much: they expand a little, they contract a little. The true role of muscles is to provide strength, support, and movement. The elasticity in your body comes from the **collagen**-rich fascial network, which can lengthen and recoil, bend and move, and which surrounds, supports, and weaves its way through a whole muscle and each individual fiber within that muscle. How much fascia stretches depends very much on the weave and direction of it and which layer is in question, as there are many types of fascia in the body. Stretching is as much about the nervous system as the tissue layer. The nerves are constantly collaborating with the rest of the body, controlling and activating sensation, communicating about the safety of any particular move or stretch. These messages are far-reaching, traveling along the many branches of the nerve tree that innervate the muscles far and wide.

In Thai medical theory, nerves are classified as Sên, which, as we have seen, are pathways of movement in the body. The nerves are Earth element, but the movement that occurs through them, the transmitting of messages, is

Wind element. So, when stretching the tissue layer, by default the Sên are also being activated and stimulated. Each nerve is also surrounded by its own fascial (**myelin**) sheath, which communicates if the message of touch is hard, fast, slow and so on. This sends a message about the type of touch it has received to specific areas of the brain for processing.

The nervous system also has a big role to play in sending messages to motor nerves within muscles. If it senses danger, the muscles will engage to prevent any injury occurring. This clarifies the importance of skillful application of pressure and techniques, always working within the limits of the body to ensure that the muscles remain relaxed. If the body's limit is over-stepped, the muscles will receive a message from the nervous system to decelerate any further lengthening to prevent injury, tear, or damage to the tissues involved.

When and How Does Someone Need to be Stretched?

As a rule of thumb, a person needs stretching when they are stiff and immobile. It is easy to spot these people, as they are unlikely to be able to touch their toes. In this scenario the structures are tight.

Someone who has tense muscles but lots of range will benefit from other techniques that address the *feeling* of tension but without further increasing their flexibility. Manual therapy techniques such as deep compressions, beating, forearm rolling and so on will be beneficial, as they will get in deep but without activating more stretch or range. A muscle *can* be long and flexible, yet might feel tense.

Side note: To clarify – tight muscles benefit from stretching. Tense muscles do not need stretching but respond well to deep pressure techniques.

In Thai massage, stretching *may* form *part* of a treatment, but there are times when it is not indicated at all. For example, if someone has agitated Wind element, this would be a time to avoid moving that person around too much, especially with lots of stretches that would cause chaos in an already Windy person. This is because, if someone is naturally Windy or has agitated Wind, then they will already feel slightly chaotic and ungrounded, and more movement will further exacerbate this state.

If Fire element is out of balance, stretching is not necessary, but if you are going to perform some stretches, they will need to be applied long, strong, and deep. Fire often needs to be calmed and this approach to stretching a Fiery person will have this effect.

Twisting and squeezing stretches work best if Water element is out of balance (Fig. 14.3). Imagine a sponge filled with water and how it needs twisting and squeezing to release the fluid. Respecting and acknowledging the integrity of physical structure and combining this with an understanding of elemental imbalance is important for optimum benefit to be achieved in a session.

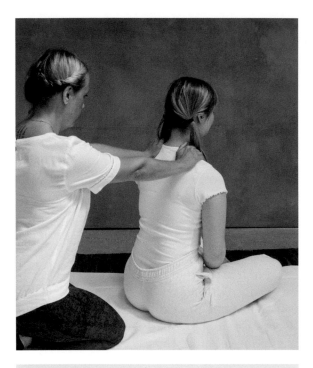

Fig. 14.3
Squeezing the second layer, rehydrating tissue and releasing bound-up tissue.

What is the Stretching Goal in Thai Massage?

In a word – hydration! And it is *movement* that hydrates the tissues in the body. Hands-on manual therapy can create movement in the body. Squeeze a muscle and imagine all the fluid being wrung out like a sponge; as it is released, the tissue fills back up with fresh fluid, hydrating it. Forearm rolling and gliding are examples of manual therapy techniques that move the fluid in that tissue. Stretch a muscle group and good juicy feelings come from movement lubricating the tissue.

Remember that stretching during Thai massage is *not* for reaching ideal flexibility, but rather to address the tissue layer so that tight or bound-up muscles or adhesions can become softer, more malleable, and more fluid. Perhaps it is helpful to think about babies and how soft and juicy their bodies are naturally, how easily they can move and bend comfortably, able to put their toes in their mouths with curious exploration of their body. They are not bound-up, tense, or tight; they are fluid and at ease, enjoying the experience of their body.

When the fascia, muscle, and soft tissues are healthier and hydrated, it allows Wind element (movement) to flow unobstructed through the underlying Sên (vessels, nerves, lymph, blood). This is the primary goal of releasing this layer. Imagine a bound-up, hard, and immobile muscle that has nerves and vessels within it: how can these smaller structures function if they too are constricted?

The Sên are physical pathways of movement in the body. When they can function properly, there is a surge of beneficial physiological changes, with the body acting as one whole ubiquitous continuation. When stretching a body, there really is no separation from one structure to another, from the core to the skin. There is an ocean of movement happening each time you stretch out an arm: the spine, organs, vessels, and leg – they all move too, ebbing and flowing with each and every part.

Stretching and Hypermobility

When someone is hypermobile and there is not enough stability in their joints, it could be that they have amplified Wind element and depleted Earth. Remember that the quality of

Earth is stable. In these cases, there are "old-style" stretches that stabilize rather than creating space by compressing the two structures closer to each other (Fig. 14.4). If there is no movement – that is, the muscles are stiff – one could say this is amplified Earth (hard tissue) and depleted Wind.

> Side note: There are sixteen old-style stretches in total, which form the basis of a lot of the Thai massage stretches known today. They also include many stabilizing stretches in which the space between two joints is compressed.

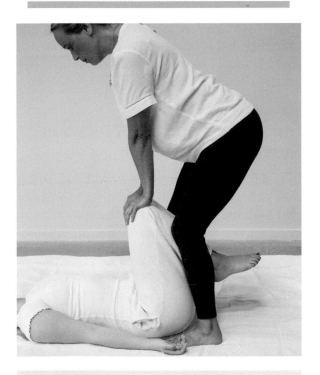

Fig. 14.4
An example of an old-style stretch.

How to Apply "Stretch"

The integrity of structure needs to be respected, which means not forcing the body to do something it does not need, or to go where it is not good for it. Keep it simple; let go of ego and an end goal.

Having the insight to know when not to perform stretches and when the "bite" (or limit) has been reached is key. This means concentrating on what you can *feel* happening, what the body you are working on is telling you, so that the stretch is appropriate and within safe limits for each individual.

> Side note: Be present with a focused mind, connected to your sense of touch, as lack of concentration can cause harm.

Each person who lies on the mat will have lived uniquely in their body, and each body expresses a different story. What someone does or does not do throughout their life, how much they express themselves, how open and how active they are, all have a direct effect on their structural integrity and capacity for movement. Understanding this is essential in informing a practitioner how to proceed with moving their client's body. It is only with time, practice, and instruction that it becomes natural to use touch to sense the precise place each limb should be moved to and for how long to hold it there. Be willing to learn, practice, and develop this aspect in yourself through receiving and giving touch.

Side note: This is something to ponder: observe the non-verbal narrative that the body expresses if you look closely at the whole person. Can someone who has emotionally closed down their heart to protect themselves still reach out their arm or leg easily? Is it the energy of the closed heart that is preventing full movement?

Another consideration is that a client's core element indicates how much of a stretch or pressure they will like. A typical Windy person will not like too much stretching, while a typical Watery person will find deep stretches or pressure painful (and bruising is more likely to occur), but they will benefit from twists. I also notice that the core element of the practitioner can influence how a massage is carried out. A Fiery therapist will get in there deeper and quicker than a watery type. This is something else to look out for – make sure your practice is not too heavily influenced by your own treatment preferences.

Stretching should be done in stages, as this mimics the recoil ability of the fascia. To do this, the first stretch of any one sequence should be to a point of minimal resistance, followed by each subsequent stretch being taken a fraction further. At no point should clients feel they are being forced or experience pain or discomfort. Each stretch should feel good as it becomes progressively deeper and the body opens up to the particular movement. When a treatment is given in this way, little by little the tissues start to release, relax, and let go; space is created. In between each of the stretches, the limb or body part should be slightly released from the stretch, allowing time for the tissue to contract and rest.

This type of stretching is called assisted progressive stretching and it allows for both the expansion and contraction of the fascial matrix. When the recipient is taken into the first stretch, it should be released only halfway back before the movement is repeated. It should then be released halfway back again, before being taken into a third stretch, then released fully. At this point, the stretch can be held longer or the practitioner can start the next technique. By only releasing the stretch halfway, it is much less work for the practitioner, more flowing for the client, and for both keeps the attention focused on the technique or stretch being applied. Working in this way means that the move feels much more effective and controlled.

Stretching and the Nervous System

In someone who is particularly stiff and inflexible, pain or restriction is usually an indicator that the nervous system is limiting movement due to it being unfamiliar or potentially dangerous.

Side note: All pain is an output of the brain and central nervous system.

If the body has not experienced a particular movement for a while, there may be a low tolerance to that movement and the nervous system will put out a red alert warning. Even though, during a Thai massage, the movements are applied and passive, there is still conscious awareness and the nervous system is active (unlike under anesthesia, where one could apply full or increased range without the nervous system firing up as protection).

When massaging an inflexible client, there is a need to apply a slow-build message to the nervous system through a considered application of touch. Work within comfortable range, easing into each movement in order for a "safe" message to be conveyed to the brain along the neural pathways. It may be that, over a period of weeks or months of treatments and regular and varied movement in their day-to-day life, they regain some of their ability to move into new positions or their range improves. During the massage, their stiffness will initially prevent many movements from being safe to perform. This is due to their body not having moved into these positions for many years and so the fascial lay-down now prevents them doing so. It is a "use it or lose it" situation, with the nervous system being the controller of what happens. When each layer of the body is cared for before any stretching, the recipient's body will already be primed for movement and will respond better to it.

However, if a client is very flexible, it may be that, while they enjoy and long for their body to be stretched (the pleasurable sensations it promotes in the body are not limited by elasticity levels in the body), it is potentially unhelpful to stretch them further, and could even be dangerous. It can be quite hard for the practitioner to feel the bite or extended range in someone who has such flexibility. When a ballet dancer, for example, is massaged, there is strength in their body, accompanied by seemingly limitless potential in the range of movement. Despite having trained their bodies this way, it is likely the "ringlets" have not returned to a natural resting length with compromised elasticity, so strengthening is key and injuries are common. Where clients are hypermobile or extremely flexible and bendy, they will benefit more from a treatment that avoids stretching altogether or uses stabilizing "old-style" stretches.

Thomas Hanna dedicated his life to researching ways for people to live a pain-free life, and developed a system of clinical somatic education. He said, "If you want to untie a knot, you must look at the cord carefully then gently undo the tangle. Yanking on the cord will only make the knot tighter."

15 Herbs, Compresses, and Infusions

Most of the knowledge of herbs used in Thai medicine comes from the Reusi of old, the medicine men and women of Thailand. They would have studied one plant for years, possibly a lifetime, experimenting with it both internally and externally. This exploration would have involved ingesting the plant – its leaves, stems, seeds, and roots. The Reusi would have tested a plant fresh and dried, with and without food, sometimes eating *only* this one plant for many days or weeks. They would have rubbed the plant on their bodies, both heated and cooled, to experience the varying effects. They would have observed and meditated on the effects on their bodies and mind, considering how the plant moved blood and Wind. They would have recorded this information so it could be shared with a wider community and taught by practitioners.

Herbs are most powerful when made into formulas. There is a historical formula with five herbs that was produced by six Reusi. Five Reusi studied one plant each, yet it was a sixth Reusi who mixed the herbs together, producing an effective formula that they then tested. This formula is called **Benjagoon**; it balances the elements, and is effective when taken as the seasons change, to prevent illness.

We can only imagine that acquiring this level of knowledge must have made the Reusi very ill at times, poisoning themselves, hallucinating, or even dying in their quest for wisdom to share with and benefit all. It is because of these explorations into the safety and efficacy of herbs that there should be deep appreciation for the Reusi of the past when working with Thai medicinal herbs.

In this book, herbs, leaves, roots, fruits, spices, and so on are all described under the heading of "herbs."

Side note: As traditional formulas for Thai herbal medicines are extremely effective, I have started producing healing balms, liniments, infusions, and compresses to use with clients, and also teach others how to make them for bodywork, steams, saunas, smokes, and scrubs. They soon become an essential part of the toolkit.

There is something so gratifying about the process of making and producing an herbal recipe that will help someone feel good. It is usually a big-time commitment, as most formulas involve pounding and crushing herbs one by one for hours. Balms and liniments require patience, as they need weeks to mature and daily turning to infuse the carrier oil with the medicinal herbal properties. Sometimes they need to be kept in the dark or heated without making them too hot. I call the making of balms a labor of love because it is time-consuming and can be heart-breaking. Many times it can go wrong: the balms end up rotting or the oil burning, the outcome being that they end up being thrown out. The hard work and expense are lost. However, every time this happens, it is part of learning and the same mistake will not be repeated.

Tastes

Five-taste systems exist in Thai medicine but for the manual therapist it is the four-taste system that is mostly used. However, for interest, here are the other taste systems:

- *Three-taste* – recipes with numerous herbs are prescribed for internal use.

- *Four-taste* – external application.

- *Six-taste* – general use of herbs in foods/cuisine.

- *Eight-taste* – formulas of herbs with an additional transporter to focus the therapeutic property of an herb to a particular area.

- *Nine-taste* – singular medicinal herbs for internal use.

Side note: Examples of transporters include alcohol, oil, urine, and camphor.

The Four Tastes

Smell is one of the most important sensory stimuli for our (twenty-six) senses and is what gives us detailed taste. Without the sense of smell, the tastes are limited to sweet, salty, and sour.

In traditional Thai medicine, the four-taste system is used to choose herbs for therapeutic and external use. (As we have seen, there are other taste-systems for internal use.) Different herbs reach different layers of the body, and are chosen for this purpose. Herbs in compresses, balms, and liniments are intended to work generally on the first four layers of the body but not the organs.

Side note: Organs are treated with internal formulas, food as medicine, and a specialized compress formula that penetrates to the viscera.

Herbs, Compresses, and Infusions

Side note: The science and use of herbs for healing are complex, and comprehensive instruction from a teacher is necessary for safe practice. Despite the ingredients being natural, it is essential to see herbs as medicine and to know that they, too, can have contraindications.

The list of herbs below is not exhaustive. For a more in-depth list and information about the taste systems, see the Resources section at the back of the book. I have tried to list herbs that are more readily available in the West, rather than giving a full list of herbs for each taste. A comprehensive list can be found in Pierce Salguero and Nephyr Jacobsen's *Thai Herbal Medicine* (see Resources).

The taste for the skin layer is spicy and hot. Herbs such as betel leaf, black pepper, calamus, camphor, plai, clove, galangal, ginger, garlic, and zedoary all work on this layer and penetrate to the deeper layers, helping to disperse stagnation, soothe muscles, and reduce pain. Herbs such as nutmeg, star anise, cinnamon, nutgrass, mint, and lemongrass are warming but not spicy, and are usually listed as aromatic and pungent. Aromatic and pungent tastes are good for calming the mental Winds; the more floral of these are best for this.

Side note: Floral waters such as jasmine, rose, and sandalwood are calming to the heart and mind (known in Thai medicine as the heart-mind).

Astringent herbs such as nutmeg, safflower, tamarind leaves, turmeric, pomegranate rind, papaya seed and mangosteen rind address the skin layers and the superficial fascia, the layer that is tightly adhered to the skin. The superficial fascia is a spongy, watery layer and the astringent herbs help to draw out dampness and assist in detoxification.

The third layer of the body (Sên) and the deeper layers of tissue (deep fascia) in the second layer are addressed by a sour taste. Herbs such as kaffir lime fruit, lime, long pepper, mace, tamarind leaves, and unripe papaya are able to penetrate to the deep fascia, clearing the way for Wind to move along the channels, and cleaning out blockages in the tissue and channels.

Salty taste addresses the bone (fourth layer) of the body. Sea salt, oyster shell, and coconut are used (salt being most common). Salt is added to all compresses, apart from those made for pregnant women (for whom it is contraindicated). It is the ingredient that gives the compresses their ability to retain heat. Salt is a healing substance for wounds and softens hard tissue, while also being helpful for joint inflammation. Salt is beneficial for drawing moisture and is therefore excellent postpartum and for conditions involving water retention.

Sweet taste involves herbs such as rice, pumpkin, milk, longan, licorice, honey, ginger, golden shower, and fennel. This is the taste that calms nerves that are over-exerting themselves, embedded into the tissue layer.

The properties of cooling herbs are self-explanatory: they cool, reduce inflammation, and calm Fire element conditions such as rashes and fevers. They include angelica, coriander, menthol, aloe, white clay, butterfly pea, and borneol.

Bitter is a taste that is purifying and targets the health of blood in the channels. These herbs include Asiatic pennywort, basil, calamus, coriander, galangal, and durian.

Side note: Camphor is a carrier and is used in many recipes and formulas, whether internal or external, as it allows the therapeutic effects of the other herbs to be activated. In the taste system it is classified as heating. Internally, it is toxic and is an adrenal stimulant; if ingested, it should be in tiny amounts as part of a healing and necessary formula.

Contraindications

Herbal formulas can cause reactions and skin irritations. Always check to see if the recipient is allergic to any roots, leaves, nuts, seeds, grasses and so on before applying herbs. Despite being natural, they can still be an irritant or trigger allergies. It is important for the compresses to be treated as medicinal. If in any doubt about using them, it is best to leave them out.

Hot compresses should not be applied to areas of inflammation, rashes, or burns. Instead, you should heat the compresses and leave them to cool in the fridge, and then apply them cold to the area.

Discovering Compresses

Many years ago, when I was studying in Bangkok, I went for a massage and for the first time experienced hot compresses applied to my body. It was a wonderful, completely unexpected, and much appreciated addition to the more regular Thai massage I was having each day. I was so relaxed at the end of the session it was ridiculous. The practitioner had used steam-heated balls to massage my body, both through my clothes and directly on my skin. He massaged me quite deeply with them, but the heat was so nurturing that it all felt amazing.

Leaving the massage and walking in a dreamy state towards the bus stop through the busy city streets, I started to notice that some people were laughing when they looked at me. Feeling somewhat disconcerted, I looked down at myself and realized that my skin was in fact bright yellow.

Intrigued, I returned the following day to find out more about the herbal compresses, and asked the practitioner to teach me about them, which he did. It was turmeric and plai (cassumunar ginger) that had turned me the color of the sun. It transpired that he had used a wonderful concoction of many herbs, which was steam-heated and then used for massage. I spent the next two days with him learning how to make the compresses and discovering the medicinal properties of the herbs and how to use them in a massage.

I was intrigued as I watched him throwing handfuls of ingredients one at a time into a big mortar and then pounding them to a pulp with a pestle. Once the ingredients were beaten sufficiently, he mixed them together and scooped up a handful, placed them in the center of a muslin square, pulled all the corners together, and twisted it (Fig. 15.1). He tied a piece of string around the top and wound it round, making a handle that would hold it together in a neat, compact bundle. This was then placed into a huge rice steamer and he repeated this to make the rest of the batch, using up all the ingredients.

Hot herbal compresses are probably the most-used and beneficial tools a practitioner can have. There is nothing not to love about them. They become an extension of the practitioner's hands and can be applied in multiple ways to

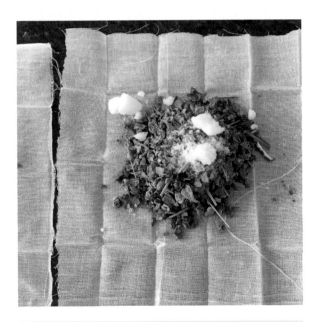

Fig. 15.1
Herbal compress ingredients before tying up the bundles.

warm the skin and work into the subsequent layers. The heat, the use of medicinal herbs in the form of tools such as compresses and balms, and massage combine to provide a nourishing, supportive, and deeply therapeutic treatment with barely any effort for the practitioner and, depending on the formula, are safe for all.

Medicinal Compresses

Herbs, roots, leaves, flowers, and minerals are the ingredients used in compresses. Various combinations are made into recipes that have properties that are penetrating, releasing, relaxing, healing, and soothing, working four layers of the body in one go. There are not many tools in a practitioner's toolkit that do such remedial work so easily. There are also special formulas that address the organs (fifth layer) directly.

The compresses are steam-heated, filling the room with wonderful smells. Inhaling this medicinal steam is beneficial for both practitioner and recipient. It is good for relieving congestion in the sinuses, lungs, and respiratory tract. The herbs are transferred from the bundles, through the clothes or cloth, via the process of conduction.

The heat of herbal compresses cares for the skin layer, using its ability to absorb as an easy way to get the medicinal properties into the body. As an organ of elimination, the skin layer is opened up by the heat and herbs. Furthermore, they penetrate into the deeper layers of the body while also calming the mental Winds with their grounding effects. Herbs come from the earth and they affect the Earth body parts.

The compresses make light and easy work for the practitioner, providing a tool for therapeutic work that does not exhaust their body. Using specific recipes, it is possible to treat many ailments and conditions safely: nature's medicine at its best.

Ready-Made Compresses

The internet has made it fairly easy to buy ready-made, generic compresses. They tend to vary in quality and ingredients, and so I suggest buying a couple to sample before buying in bulk. Open one up and look inside it to check that there are many different herbs making up the compress (in the past I have opened up compresses to find sawdust). Use the other to experiment with during massage to establish how effective it is, how long-lasting, how therapeutic. It is worth shopping around and testing out a few before going ahead with a large order. Good-quality ready-made compresses are very generalized and are useful for regular muscular tension and aches and pains. They are always warming compresses, which are contraindicated in pregnancy (see Chapter 24).

Ready-made compresses are more expensive than ones you make yourself, but it is useful to have some to hand and there are some very good generic ones available (see Resources). They are also time-efficient, as you do not need to shop around for specific herbs or spend time crushing or chopping the ingredients.

Making compresses is a really satisfying process. It is a good idea to make a recipe in big batches and store in an airtight container. Have a few pieces of muslin or cotton fabric on the go that can be washed and reused. It is helpful to have a warming recipe, a drying compress for joints, and an energy-boost formula at the ready (all recipes can be found in *Thai Herbal Medicine*). There are compresses specifically for pregnant women, and others can be tailored to individual client's needs.

You can use dried *or* fresh herbs, but choose one of these and do not mix them, as this does not work and you will find the compresses go off quickly. Fresh and dried herbs also steam at varying speeds, causing them to release their healing properties differently, which is another reason not to mix them.

Compresses made with fresh ingredients also feel different to the recipient, with a wetter and softer texture. They are not as good for doing deep physical work (although the herbs still penetrate deeply). They heat much more quickly: five to ten minutes should be sufficient.

A blend can be chosen carefully to suit each individual, and can be supportive to ease many complaints such as a cough or cold, soothe tense muscles, help the joints, release nerves, increase energy, reduce water retention, speed up healing, aid pregnant women, and much more. Herbal compresses can be used hot, cold, or dry-heated, although it is most common to steam-heat them and use them hot.

The use of these herbal compresses is an example of how two branches of the Thai medical system (physical therapy and herbal medicine) are combined.

Hot Steamed Compresses

Hot compresses are often used when direct pressure is too much or there is increased sensitivity. They are also employed when someone is depleted and heat is needed to open up the body, relieve muscular tension, and nourish

Wind element. They can be used to stimulate Sên, provide wonderful care for joints, and increase flexibility. They can be applied as preparation for deeper work, but are also sufficient for deep and nurturing work when a client is below par or weak.

They are also useful when time is limited. They can be placed in areas that need work but that there may not be time to address in the session. This way, the area receives attention while work is being done elsewhere. An example is placing them under the neck when working on the legs or abdomen in supine position.

Storage and Shelf Life

Compresses can normally be used four to six times over the space of two weeks before they lose their potency. A compress used on one client should not be used on another, for hygiene reasons. Even though they are boiled for long periods, which does sterilize them, it is safer practice to refrain from using a compress on more than one person. When a treatment using an herbal compress is finished, the compress should be allowed to cool, and then kept in a fridge in an airtight container. The muslin or cloth can be washed and reused. The compress can also be given to the recipient to take home and use as self-care between sessions.

Making Compresses

To make a compress you will need to crush all the ingredients one by one in a pestle and mortar. If you do not have a pestle and mortar, you can put them into a plastic bag or wrap them in a large cloth. A stick or big stone can be used to crush the contents. Pound the herbs. When each herb has been crushed so it is in small pieces (but not powdered), mix them all together, using your hands or a big spoon to do this.

You will need two muslin squares, which should measure approximately 30 cm × 30 cm (a good measurement is from elbow to fingertips square). Use both hands to scoop up a big pile of the mixture and place in the center of each fabric; bring all the edges together, making sure nothing spills out. Twist the wraps and tie up with elastic bands or string.

There are many clever ways to bind and tie the string, some of which are very fancy, but as no one ever really looks at them it is not necessary to make them look the part. You need the handle to be strong and solid, and the compress to be firm to hard. Dip both compresses a little way into water first to make them just slightly moist, and then place in an electrical steamer or rice cooker; heat for 15–30 minutes. Two old (but clean) cotton socks can be substituted if you do not have any muslin.

How to Heat Compresses

Dip the compresses in water, making sure that they are not sodden (you can wring them out if you need to). Place them in a steamer and heat for 20–30 minutes if they are dry herb, or for 10 minutes if fresh herb. If your steamer has a temperature gauge, use it at about 60–80 degrees, but test it and take care. The compresses will come out extremely hot and so you will need to have a cloth to wrap around them and/or the handle to make them easier to hold until they cool down. Initially, you may also need an extra layer with which to cover the recipient to ensure that there is more of a barrier.

If you do not have an electric steamer or rice cooker, you can put the compresses in a colander placed above a large pan of water. The compresses should not come into direct contact with the water or they will get soaked and the potency of the herbs will be lost. You will have to experiment with your timing if using this substitute method of heating as, unlike steamers which have a timer or cook/steam option, a pan of water is just going to boil and potentially dry out if not frequently topped up.

Clothing

Make sure the recipient is wearing loose, comfortable, wide-legged cotton trousers, such as Thai fisherman trousers. If you can provide a cotton top that fastens at the back, then this is ideal; otherwise ask the recipient to bring with them an old T-shirt that they do not care about (this is because some ingredients like turmeric or galangal will stain).

You will need to practice and experiment a little with these compresses to master how to use them and to make sure that when you apply them to the skin they are not too hot. Be aware that if you leave them on the body in one place for any length of time, the intensity of the temperature increases fairly quickly.

A herbal compress should be applied warm or hot to the skin until it cools down, when it should be replaced by another from the steamer.

One layer of clothes is enough to give some protection from the initial heat, but a thin cotton scarf can be useful if an extra layer is needed initially. When the compress is cooler, it can be applied directly to the skin. Check and ask for feedback regarding temperature, as people have very different sensitivities. When you are holding the compresses, they can feel very hot; this is misleading, as recipients will mostly feel the temperature as cooler than you do because they are not in constant contact with it.

Luk Prakhob

In Thailand, the technique of pressing herbal compresses to the body is known as **Luk Prakhob**.

Take a compress out of the steamer and check the temperature by pressing it against the inside of your wrist or forearm. The wrist and forearm have a thin layer of skin, so by testing the heat on this area you will have a good sense of the temperature. If the compress is too hot, you can pound it against your arm a few times, and this cools it down. You could also wrap it in an extra layer of cotton or muslin until it cools down sufficiently. If the temperature is ideal, then press the compress and roll it away from you, covering thoroughly the area you are treating.

Initially, you can work through clothes, and then when the compresses have cooled slightly they can be directly applied to the skin. As with any application of touch, you should lean in with your body weight to create some pressure. You can roll the side of the compresses around an area or down a channel. Compresses become like an extension of your hands and (with some practice) it becomes easy to feel with them what is going on in the recipient's body.

Do not leave the compresses on any one point until you are certain that the temperature is manageable.

Techniques with Compresses

If you are planning to use the compresses on specific therapy points as a treatment, then work the point over and over again but be aware at all times of how comfortable this is for the receiver as the heat can get intense; you can, of course, ask for feedback.

You can use the side of the compresses to slide them up and down the channels with firm pressure that comes from leaning, not brute strength.

The compresses can be used for:

- dragging tissue

- spreading and gliding

- deep compressions (once they have cooled) and palpation

- kneading

- beating

- rolling (the side can be used to roll up and down areas)

- point press/warm

- counterpressure (the weight of the body can be moved on to the compresses)

- traction (I use this mainly on the neck in supine).

(See Chapter 20.)

Rotate the compresses so that, as they cool, they are put back into the steamer and replaced each time with a hot one, closing the steamer lid to ensure that the steam stays hot and the water does not evaporate. Always open the steamer lid away from you and without leaning directly over it.

Directional Work

Combining the compresses with directional work increases their efficacy.

Cold Compresses

Contrary to popular belief, ice is not good for healing injuries – while it may *initially* take down the inflammation, it prevents the body's own natural healing process, by which nutrients in the blood try to reach the area to heal it. Sên, structures that are pathways of movement in the body, will not benefit from freezing temperatures that prevent the movement of blood to nourish the injury. Wind will also be inhibited rather than encouraged to an area that most needs help.

Cool or cold compresses are traditionally used, along with cooling medicinal herbs, for healing acute injuries. The medicinal properties of the herbs will support natural healing.

Prepare and heat the compresses as described earlier. Place the compresses in the fridge to cool. Cold compresses can be used like an ice-pack when there is an injury with inflammation. The cool temperature constricts blood vessels, which is particularly beneficial for swelling. A cold compress can also be useful to treat bruising, especially when the bruising accompanies inflammation. Similar to using a hot compress, it is essential that you test the compress to make sure it is not so cold that it will burn the skin when applying to the body (using compresses this cold is counterproductive to the healing process, so not advised).

Chapter 15

Dry Compresses

These are particularly good for Watery conditions such as lung congestion, colds, water retention, and postpartum disorders. They are made by placing the crushed herbs in an oven on a dish. They heat quickly (five minutes or so). When hot, they can be wrapped in a cloth or put into a sock and applied to the body area.

Ingredients for Compresses

I have chosen a few common ailments for which the use of herbs can be beneficial. If you are in doubt, please consult the recipient's doctor or health practitioner first to make sure the herbs will not adversely affect any prescription drugs, homeopathic remedies, or treatment being received.

Many of these herbs are available at the Thai or Asian supermarkets that are now widespread in big cities; others can be found online and are often available to buy in bulk; and some (such as the ever-elusive plai) are easily available only in Thailand. Shopping for herbs tends to be time-consuming and some ingredients mentioned in recipes often have to be left out as they are too hard to source.

Side note: Camphor – natural camphor – is very hard to source. Often synthetic camphor crystals are more easily available. Camphor is an important herb, as it is a carrier of the other herbs in a formula.

Salt

This should be added to compresses to affect the bone layer and to keep the heat in the compresses. Salt is drying and drawing, so should not be used in compresses during pregnancy.

Choosing Ingredients for Particular Indications

Coughs, colds, and respiratory problems

Ginger, garlic, lemongrass, cassumunar ginger (plai) or root ginger, eucalyptus leaves, peppermint leaves, cloves, and camphor crystals.

Sore and over-worked muscles

Ginger root, camphor crystals, cinnamon leaves, eucalyptus leaves, kaffir lime rind and leaves.

Headaches, anxiety, and stress

Basil leaves, peppermint leaves, jasmine flowers.

Asthma

Calamus (decongestant/treats Sên), angelica (bronchial dilator), plai (treats wind, bronchial dilator, beneficial for skin and tissue layer), cloves (opens Sên), eucalyptus, camphor (opens mucous membrane and sinuses, clears congestion, calming).

Postnatal compress

A clay pot can be heated with salt inside. As salt is drawing and drying, it is very effective in postpartum women to help their body process the extra fluids. This is specialized work and needs in-person instruction from a teacher.

Breastfeeding

Compresses encourage milk production and let-down. They are used steam-heated, and the breasts, shoulders, upper back, and legs are massaged with them.

Traditional uses

For detoxification, bruising, tissue layer, Sên layer, tightness, stagnation. Plai, galangal, ginger, turmeric, lemongrass, lime peel, tamarind leaf, salt, camphor.

Calming/soothing

Nutmeg, caraway seeds, long pepper, cardamom – dip the compress in raw or warm sesame oil and then massage directly into the skin. As the heated compress soaks up the oil, it can be redipped and reapplied.

Herbal Infusions

The herbal infusions are pleasant to drink if a sweetener such as honey, coconut blossom sugar, or maple syrup is added. They provide internal support for the physical bodywork treatments. There are many recipes, the following being the most commonly used.

1. *An infusion for opening the Sên.* This helps prepare the Sên and soften the fascia to make working the third layer possible.

2. *A post-bodywork purifying infusion.* As the name suggests, this helps support the body after deep work that has moved stagnation. It helps the body to cleanse.

3. *A kidney infusion.* This is beneficial when someone is low and functioning below par. It is supportive and nourishing for the kidneys.

4. *An infusion for the menses.* This is particularly helpful when menstruation is late or irregular.

All of these are therapeutic but (like all medicine) should be taken only when needed. For details of all recipes, see Resources.

Two Recipes

Golden Milk

This is an amazing recipe for aiding restful sleep, calming anxiety, and helping a person to feel revitalized on waking.

Although shop-bought almond milk could be used, it tends to have preservatives and other ingredients added to it, so it is more medicinal (and therefore therapeutic) to make a fresh batch.

Chapter 15

Herbal component

- Nutmeg
- Cardamom
- Saffron
- Sesame

The ingredients should be crushed and made into a powder.

To make almond milk

- Soak nuts overnight.
- Rinse and peel.
- Blend with some water.
- Put in a muslin cloth and squeeze out liquid.
- Keep refrigerated for 3–4 days.
- Add a spoonful of the powdered herbs to a cup of warmed almond milk and drink. Add honey or maple syrup to taste, if needed.

Moon Milk

- Turmeric
- Ginger
- Cinnamon
- Black pepper
- Cardamom
- Coconut oil
- Cashew or almond milk (as above)
- Additional: Hemp oil or paste. Magnesium powder

The method is the same as for Golden Milk.

Side note: While the medicine of Thailand can mostly be attributed to Reusi monks and to village doctors who would use what was available to them for healing, information would also have been exchanged during trade between one part of the country and another, or across borders, between one tribe and another. Buddhism would also have played a role in the development of medicine, as people would have talked about their experiences with herbs, much as they do today with medicine and health in general. Additionally, very simple remedies would have been used, especially in remote areas. These would include drinking urine for healing, using urine externally to soothe the skin, and mixing urine with earth for treating a snake bite.

16

Energy, Life Force, Kwan, and Death

Thai Massage is *not* an energy-based modality. I want to be sure we are really clear about this before continuing. It is very much a physical therapy (being one aspect of the physical therapy root of the medicine). The massage and bodywork are based on tangible structures and pathways of movement that occur in the body. Neither are Sên energy lines or meridians.

Despite there not being a word for "energy" in the traditional Thai medical system, I am making mention of it because the body *is* energy and any type of input – be it nutritional, touch-based, or a thought – has a direct energetic impact.

Energy

Energy is a natural phenomenon, present everywhere in life. Anything that we touch, move, or see, whether it is solid, liquid, or gas, consists of light particles that are moving towards each other, oscillating and vibrating at various speeds. At the point where the atoms and molecules are fully compressed, they become form. The body is no exception to this rule: it has many vibrating frequencies of energy, all of which combine to make up the physical body. All energy and cellular activity

happen with an exchange of electro-magnetic energy. Candace Pert, who wrote *The Molecules of Emotion* (1999), writes about the author Dr James L. Oschman's "vision of the body as a liquid crystal under tension, capable of vibrating as a number of frequencies, some in the range of visible light."

Our bodies are made of light particles conducting with water. The light, which is energy, compresses and slows down to become form. An individual's electro-magnetic field, sometimes known as their aura, is an expansion of energy. Health in human form is an uninterrupted movement of both compressed and expanding energy.

Most Eastern approaches to the body are characterized by a recognition of energy as a core aspect of health and illness: the Indian Yogic system uses prana as its energy system and chakras as energy centers, while Chinese traditional medicine has **chi** as its energy system. Ancient Western approaches to medicine also regarded illness from a similar viewpoint: that is, we have a life-force energy that affects the balance of health.

Thai medicine does not have a specific word for energy because the body, seen through a Thai lens, is identified as physical matter. However, the elements of Fire and Wind are the energetic functions of the body, which have an effect on the physical elements.

Side note: The interconnection and interdependence of everything, with no one aspect separated from the other, are also acknowledged through the five elements.

Space is the first element, the beginning of all life, and a place for all other elements to play out. If taken literally, Space is not dense or compacted; it is unobstructedness, where there are gaps between the molecules. And if there are gaps, then there must be distance between two things, and there must be an organizing force or "energy" that brings these things closer together. As everything gathers, it starts densifying.

The first form is consciousness, known as **Viññāna**. It then becomes Wind and Fire, before finally turning dense and solid as Earth and Water. The human body, its anatomy, has the same qualities of Earth and Water. Wind and Fire are our physiology; they are the less tangible and the more "energetic" of the elements.

In Thai bodywork, the less solid a condition has become, the easier it is to change because, once the dis-ease progression has really set into the physical body, it has densified and slowed down a lot. This makes it more impenetrable and therefore harder to dissipate. Earth and Water are slower and the most dense aspects of the physical body, whereas Fire and Wind are lighter and faster-moving. Touch techniques can help assist the body (Earth and Water) to repair and disperse stagnation through the warming up of those tissues (Fire), which creates movement (Wind) and Space in the physical body again.

Death

Let's look at this from a different and non-Thai perspective for a moment. We will take death as the starting point and look at things in reverse; in doing this, we start with form.

In observing a dead body, we first see that it has been released from animation. If we watched for longer, we would see it go through the process of decomposition and would notice the following: the body undoing itself, breaking down, releasing and dispersing what made it. It would start to liquefy and then would give off gases. These gases would eventually become ethers, and then such rarefied ethers that their speed and frequency would be too fast to see, feel, and/or smell. There would be space between the atoms and molecules. What would be left would be the skeleton, a substance that was once a liquid that calcified to bone, in order for all our other liquid (soft) tissues to have something to which to attach. The skeleton is the end result of all that we are, and it (bone) has an astonishing ability to regenerate (Fig. 16.1).

Many times, I have heard stories of people who have been with someone during their last moments or the minutes leading up to their death. There is a very particular energy during this precious time. To those with awareness of such things, the spirit or soul reveals itself in pure form, sometimes slipping away from the physical body before the heart stops.

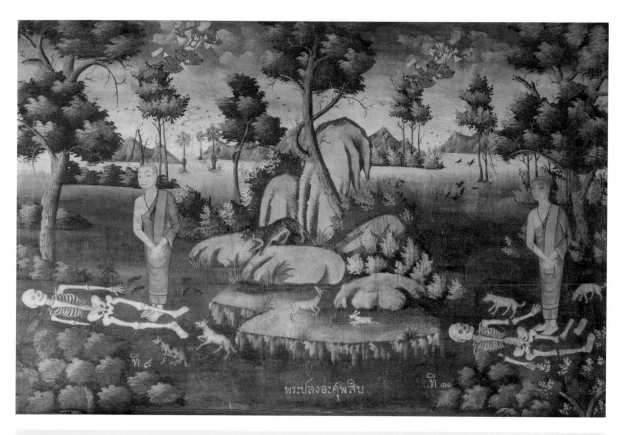

Fig. 16.1
The Skeleton is Earth element and the last to disperse into the ethers. By special permission of Tim Bewer.

However, it is most common for people to notice that, for some time after the person has stopped breathing and life has slipped away, the energy of that person is still there – their soul, or spirit. My sister and I experienced this when our grandmother died. We sat with her for a long time after she took her last breath, and two hours or so later we knew she had gone. The soul hangs around, dissipating into the ethers long after the body ceases to function.

We experienced this again more recently when our father died. We watched him as he took his last breath. This breath was an exhalation, ending the cycle of breathing. We breathe in as we are born and breathe out as our final letting go and release of this life.

At the other end of the spectrum of life, it is well known that anyone attending a birth is aware of a very particular energy or life force. In both instances (birth and death), the

Chapter 16

energy is fast-moving, not dense and slow, but closer to Space. It is the energy of becoming or unbecoming.

One of the most powerful experiences I have ever had was in an embalming suite during a dissection. A woman had died and had left her body to science. There is only a short window between death and preservation of tissue, so she had not long arrived. I saw her when she was being prepared for the embalming procedure. I knew at that very instant that her spirit had not yet left her body. She was not a cadaver, but a dead woman whose soul was still present; the difference is worlds apart. I placed my hands on her warm skin and I sat with her until her spirit left her body. I deeply loved this woman, whom I only ever met when she was dead. I will never forget her; she was a generous teacher. She provided an extraordinary and intimate experience, and cemented in my mind forever the existence of Kwan – life force, energy.

Kwan

Kwan, loosely translated as life force, life spirit, or soul, is an important aspect of Thai anatomy. The thirty-two body parts that make up the physical body (twenty from Earth element and twelve from Water; see Chapter 3) each have their own essential element, their own life force, called Kwan, which is directly connected to the physical body (there are therefore thirty-two body parts and thirty-two Kwan).

Consider how the body as a whole organizes itself, holds itself together, communicates throughout the whole system, regenerates, breaks and then mends, and somehow innately knows how to do this – this can be attributed to Kwan.

While Kwan is connected to the body, its nature is fragile, complex, and intricate. It has a lightness to it, and is easily affected by external forces. Kwan is the life force that connects the mind and the body.

Thais believe strongly in all kinds of spirits. These beliefs interweave throughout the whole of Thai culture and tradition. Spirits exist everywhere, whether in the body, on a piece of land, or in a house or tree. They can cause disruption or ill health, make a piece of land become less healthy, or cause a tree to die. Because of the Thais' strong belief in spirits, they are often seen as the primary cause when something goes wrong, and there are many people who acknowledge that it is always important to make sure the spirits are looked after and respected. There are miniature spirit houses outside every building, home, and office, which acknowledge the spirits that resided there first (Fig. 16.2). The spirits in these houses are kept happy with offerings so that they do not cause trouble.

Kwan is seen as a spirit that brings things to life, but it can easily be broken or harmed, or even lost or stolen. There are special ceremonies for reclaiming or mending broken Kwan. Family members might sing a healing Kwan song, or make supportive and nourishing food, and will generally help the affected person to rest and recuperate in order to help the Kwan to come back into their body.

As Westerners who are not raised with spirit traditions, it is often hard to grasp the nature of Kwan fully. In Thailand, it is part of normal everyday life; everyone knows about it and *everything* has Kwan, whether it is a tree, car, building, boat, piece of land, or animal. It is common to see trees with multiple colored strings tied

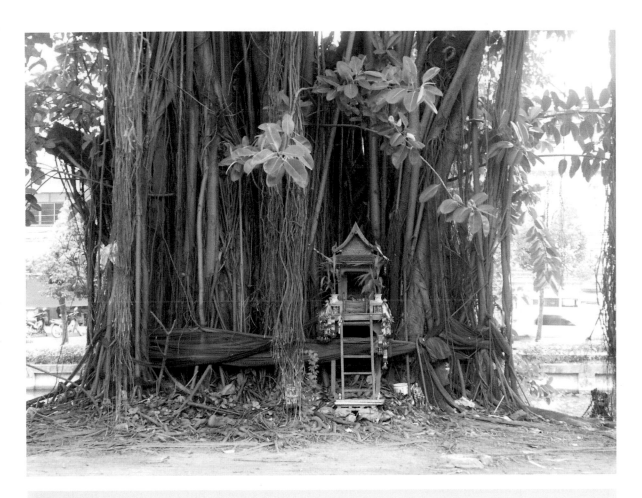

Fig. 16.2
A Bodhi tree with Kwan strings tied to it and a spirit house. By special permission of Pierce Salguero.

around them all over Thailand. These are Kwan strings, which help their Kwan stay with them. If a tree is damaged in strong winds or looks weak, it will be held up with sticks to support it and help it regain strong Kwan.

Humans also wear Kwan strings at special times in their lives and are given them at pivotal moments. The strings are tied at the wrist (which is where the pulse is used as diagnosis of the elements). They can be attached by a monk as a blessing, to a newborn child, whose Kwan is seen as fragile and not yet fully attached to their physical body. They are also tied to students' wrists by teachers at the end of a course of study to symbolically hold their new knowledge to them and to recognize the

125

beginning of a journey. Other examples would be starting school for the first time, getting married, taking the precepts, making a commitment to Buddhist studies, or even after a child has a first haircut.

Someone who has been through a trauma is seen as having damaged Kwan. Often, in times of trauma, it is easy to see that there is something that has changed in the person, that they appear vulnerable or weakened. At other times, we can be lackluster and have no drive or zest for life; these qualities indicate that there could be an issue with Kwan. Kwan can easily be harmed and may even leave the body entirely. Practitioners of Thai bodywork need to understand at a basic level that Kwan exists, as it helps to explain the importance of spirit in Thai medicine and the fact that some illnesses might not be purely physical.

Often, in the West, if we cannot see something or have tangible and constant proof in front of us that something exists, we have a hard time believing in it. We put most value in what we can see. In terms of the body, we can easily forget what created it, forget about Space and a gathering force. We become "body-centered" and "form-focused," seeing ourselves as solid objects, and often forgetting (or completely lacking) appreciation for the totality of ourselves, which includes spirit, life force, and the electro-magnetic field.

Side note: I am mixing up some Western concepts with Thai theory here, as I think it helps those of us with Western minds to understand an area we are not generally raised to pay much attention to.

Thai element theory, Buddhist philosophy, and quantum physics all regard the importance of Space in the becoming of everything, including form. Space element *is* the expansiveness of nothing and everything; it is where there is most potential. It is the negative space around us, which defines us as all that we are, in relation to all we are not. Space is expansive and pervasive, and because of this it is a place where all the other elements can exist.

Intuition

How is it that we can know that someone is feeling a certain way by looking at them? We have antennae that pick up signals from their energetic field. During Thai massage, we are doing this all the time, tapping into subtle frequencies, our personal vibration and resonation meeting and often mirroring the receiver's. There is silent, non-verbal yet powerful communication that can happen through touch.

It is not uncommon for people to mention being able to see a slight or faint glow around a person; this is a dense form of energy, often known as the etheric body, which is the liquid nervous system. But often people try to "see" energy; they are consciously looking for it, and in doing so they miss it. To be able to see, feel, or sense the subtle energy of the body needs an altered approach. In the same way as you might see or sense something in your peripheral vision, or know that someone is close behind you, there is a definite awareness of something, yet it is intangible. If you look directly at it or put conscious awareness on it, you can see only one perspective, which is form. To feel energy, you must work in a slightly altered state of mind; it is not possible to work with or sense energy with a very conscious mind-set. Thai bodywork and massage have their effects predominantly on the physical body, so practitioners do not need to "feel energy" to perform effective therapeutic work. Yet there are many practitioners who also have a sense of something else, and being open to this can be illuminating. The process of reflection and staying curious opens us up to these more subtle aspects of awareness.

The body absorbs the water we drink, the air we breathe, and the food we eat, all of which nourish us, contribute to our health, and give us energy, but the body is not created from water, food, or air. These are external energetic factors that are not part of human makeup. The naturally occurring energy or life force is what creates our form. The body then processes many energetic exchanges to function: that is, the food we eat gives us energy and it takes digestive energy to break it down. We also have other types of energy, such as chemical, electrical, kinetic, metabolic, digestive, and muscular. Each process in the creation or experience of life is created by something that came before it. Claude Bernard, a French physiologist and scientist from the 1800s, said "genes create structures, but the genes do not control them; the vital force does not create structures, the vital force directs them".

The body is approximately 65 percent liquid, and is affected by external forces such as the Moon and Sun, and the natural rhythms and cycles of life. All movements of energy, including thoughts, feelings, and touch, also influence the body and its functionality. The mind, body, and soul are one, not separated or segmented from *any* aspect of the whole.

"The energy of the mind is the essence of life."

Aristotle, 2011

Vibration

A Japanese scientist, Masaru Emoto, proved that thoughts impact on our biological makeup. He spoke words to water, or put words around a container that had water in it. He used photography under a microscope to capture images of the water as it crystallized and became frozen. From this, it was possible to see that the water molecules reacted to each word (Fig. 16.3). He found that negative words such as "hate" or

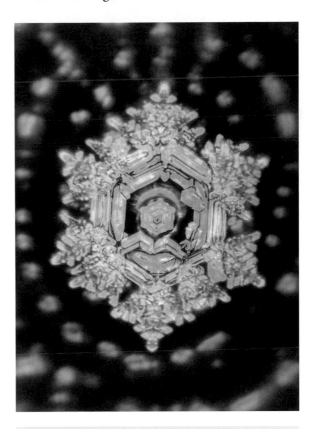

Fig. 16.3
Buddhist chants spoken to water. From the book *Hidden Messages in Water*. By special permission of Masaru Emoto.

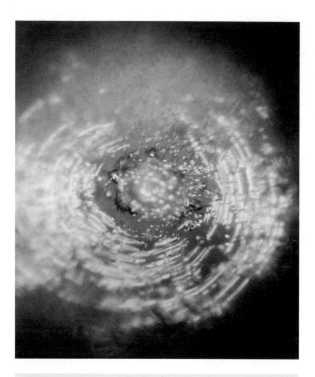

Fig. 16.4
The words "you fool," spoken to water. From the book *Hidden Messages in Water*. By special permission of Masaru Emoto.

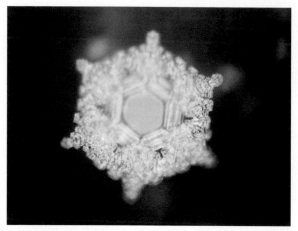

Fig. 16.5
Words of "love and compassion" spoken to water. From the book *Hidden Messages in Water*. By special permission of Masaru Emoto.

phrases such as "you fool" (Fig. 16.4) made fragmented, ugly, and distorted structures of the water's crystallized formations, while words like "love" or "peace" did the opposite and made beautiful, visually pleasing, and more symmetrical shapes (Fig. 16.5). His work proves that thoughts,words, and intention have an impact on physical form.

A word has the ability to be very healing and very harming. You can make someone feel amazing by saying one word of kindness or acknowledgement, and yet another word that is negative, disempowering, or unkind can do the complete opposite.

It is very important to remember this when you talk with clients. Their body will respond to your words, and the resonation of a word is extremely powerful.

This is a good time to mention again the importance of a daily Wai Kru as a self-care practice when giving treatments. Chanting sacred words in a deep, resonant voice before the day starts gives the practitioner an embodied experience of the sacred words and strong intentional tools for healing. It helps us have a healthy mind-set, which impacts our own health and that of our clients.

This chant forms a very small part of a daily Wai Kru. It is also chanted all over the world, by so many people at any one given time, that it has an extra power to it. You will never be chanting it alone:

NAMO TASSA BHAGAVATO ARAHATO SAMMĀ SAMMBUDDHASSA

PART 3

The Practice

17 The Art of Consultation

Before we start looking at the consultation, I would like to mention something a teacher once said to me.

There are three types of people:

- those who get better with or without treatment or medicine

- those who do not get better with or without treatment or medicine

- those who get better with *medicine* and treatment.

It is this third group of people who need to see us.

The consultation part of the session is crucially important; in fact, it is where the healing process begins. Listening to the narrative is illuminating, yet is often overlooked or rushed through to reach the hands-on work. There are huge therapeutic benefits in slowing down this aspect of the treatment. It is important to create a safe environment for a client to be heard and to have space to voice their history, thoughts, feelings, and beliefs. The consultation is often like piecing together a puzzle of the client's life and habits to figure out how best to help,

and to give guidance about making changes their usual ways, especially if these are causing imbalance and pain.

Side note: In my experience, people do not always make the best choices for themselves in regard to their health, and when asked about it, they lie. They do not want to say that they are eating rubbish instead of fresh foods, taking little or no exercise, or staying up too late. They often say what they think you want them to say, so keep this in mind and do not judge.

There are many considerations for a practitioner, and the variables can alter treatment choices. Treatment will depend on your level of training, the tools in your toolkit, your level of experience, and much more.

Each session starts with a consultation, which is an art in itself and contains many paths that can be taken. In this chapter, I analyze the process to give you an idea of what you might be looking for and how to use your findings to inform your bodywork.

Chapter 17

Observations and Assessment

Doctors of traditional medicine would use many observations and tools for diagnosis. These might include reading the pulse, looking at the tongue, and studying and smelling the stools of the recipient, as well as looking at seasonal, elemental, and planetary influence, age, karma, spirits, daily habits, and much more, to ascertain the treatment needed.

We do not necessarily need to smell stools to decide how to work with clients for the purposes of therapeutic massage, but it is helpful to ask clients what their stools smell and look like, especially if they have digestive problems or are low in energy. This gives an indication of how the food is being broken down and how many nutrients are being absorbed; if they have bloating or pain, the reason will often be obvious when you know more about their stools. Digestive health and gut health are important for diagnosis. How we digest is related to Fire element, how we eliminate is related to Water element, and how food moves through our digestive tract is related to Wind element.

Engaging our sense of smell and listening carefully are also useful skills during the consultation. Sometimes, we can smell the client: they may be sweaty (fresh or old), rancid, toxic, fresh, clean, sweet, and so on, and these qualities all provide clues about their general health. Listen to how they talk about what is happening in their lives. Are they loud, quiet, unsure, fearful, or anxious? Does their voice sound strong or weak?

What is their skin tone and color? Deane Juhan, in *Jobs Body* (2003), describes the skin as "the surface of the brain," and as the most superficial of layers, it demonstrates many deeper and underlying problems. Just think how the skin reddens with embarrassment, exposing a hidden thought or feeling. Dryness could indicate a lack of hydration or agitated Wind element. Oiliness could be caused by a Fire imbalance or hormonal problem. Puffiness indicates that Water element is agitated and that the body is not moving fluids through the lymphatic system quickly enough (lymph is Sên). Is the skin being used to eliminate impurities that are usually purged through feces and urine?

How much light is in the eyes, those gateways to the soul? Their brightness and the overall look in someone's eyes are illuminating. They are often a real communicator of mood and health.

I always observe my clients as they walk into the room. I might even ask them to walk up and down to see how they move. The physical body is often a very clear indicator of a person's mental state. Someone who is unhappy is very unlikely to walk into the room looking larger than life and confident, with their head raised. A client who is feeling wonderful, happy, and at ease will not be stooping, shrinking, or walking in a meek and mild manner. Someone who has a very awkward, unbalanced gait is not very likely to be feeling stable. Do they walk in a comfortable way? Do they stand upright or look as if the weight of the world is on their shoulders? Do they walk with their whole foot on the ground? Do their head and neck lead the way? Do their bony landmarks and joints appear normal? What happens when you compare one side to the other, and what information might that be giving you about function, movement patterns, and mobility?

I also spend some time looking at a client's range of motion in various joints in their body. As joints are often problematic areas, it helps establish what work might need to be done. If the client has a shoulder problem, I will ask them to extend their arm forwards, sideways, and behind. I make sure they do not do anything painful and watch how their whole body moves while they perform the task. It provides many clues about which muscles are involved in their movements and where the areas of restriction might be. I may also ask the client to repeat these movements while they are seated, to compare the range of motion with standing. All of this helps to build up a picture of their restrictions.

Questions for the Consultation

As a practitioner, the following are areas you might ask about in the consultation or might need to figure out yourself. They should be used as a springboard, and are not a definitive list because the consultation can take many different paths. Confidence comes from years of experience, study, and work with many people.

It is helpful to establish the recipient's core element constitution (CEC; see Chapter 5), as this tells you about the level of pressure they might like and what is best for them in regard to the bodywork you will provide. It also gives an indication of disease tendencies and predispositions.

The phase of life that they are currently in is also relevant. At different ages, certain elements are stronger than others, and it gives you a clearer picture if you know how the elements play out at various times.

What condition or problem is a person presenting with? (Each person will experience whatever they are suffering with differently, which is why it is important to listen to the individual describe their experience rather than being caught up with a Western diagnosis.)

Which elements are currently playing up and need balancing? (This could be showing itself on a physical level, an emotional level, or both.)

What is bothering them most? (There may be an acute injury, back pain, stiffness, weakness, and so on.) This question often leads to another important one: do you want me to work carefully around this area because it feels weak and vulnerable, or would you like me to get in there and work it deeply to release it?

How does the client sleep (at what time of night are they waking, how rested are they in the morning, is sleep disrupted by the mind being too alert or the body in pain and so on)? Time of day is linked to elements being at their strongest (see Chapter 11). Find out if they wake rested and refreshed.

The digestive system says a lot about a person, as it tells you whether food is being absorbed properly, whether they are choosing foods that are nourishing or depleting, and how quickly it goes through their digestive tract. How often they defecate, and the color, smell, and texture of their feces are useful pieces of information.

What do they like to eat and when? What do they crave? Do they eat mainly cooked or raw foods, processed or fresh? How much do they move their body and exercise? (These are not the same thing.)

How is their energy? Do they have times of day that are better or worse? Do they feel as if they have vitality?

Do they have any scar tissue, or have they had any accidents or surgery? If so, how long ago? What does the scar feel like to them? Do they touch it? How do they feel, if so?

With women, ask about their menstrual cycle. How old were they when it started/ stopped? When did they become peri-menopausal? Find out what a normal period cycle is for them. What is the color of the blood, and is it clotty, bright, or dark? Is there pain or breast tenderness?

Ask about childhood vaccinations or illnesses, as these indicate immune health.

Does the client suffer from regular headaches or migraines? Are these cyclical, hormonal, or tension headaches? Where do they occur? Ask them to describe them to you.

Some helpful questions I frequently ask include the following:

- What is it you need help with?

- Are you in pain?

- What does it prevent you doing and when do you notice it?

- Is it better or worse for movement?

- What does it feel like to you? Can you describe the pain to me?

- How long has it been going on? Did you injure yourself?

- Can you point to where it is most painful?

- Does the pain radiate up, down, or across from this area?

- If we were to use a pain scale, with 1 as feeling barely anything and 10 as absolute agony, where would you rate it right now? How about when you move/sit/stand/walk? (This is called having a "marker" and should be referred back to as treatments progress.)

- How would you describe your emotional state?

- Are you stressed or under a lot of pressure at the moment?

- How does this affect you?

- Can you tell me more about this?

All these responses should be noted down in the client file, as you can then check back in subsequent appointments.

A practitioner must be able to draw on their experience and knowledge, and be able to listen to hear what *is* and *is not* being said when the consultation is under way. This invisible and unspoken information is often sensed or intuited, and this is a technique I focus on developing with students in class. Sometimes, a tone of voice or a look in the eye can be enough to direct the plan for the session. These are often so subtle that the practitioner must be highly perceptive or experienced.

The consultation part of the session is illuminating, especially if the questions are direct and focused, and lead to more questioning. It is the questions asked, and the client's introspection, that are most important.

There is an art to the consultation process. It is a space during which clients should feel they can both open up and start to unravel what is going on internally for them. When they verbalize what is going on, there is a conscious acknowledgement of thoughts, feelings, and physical sensations. It means really taking notice of themselves.

If a client is in pain, I will often ask how it is affecting their life. They will know exactly what the impact is on their usual daily functioning. For example, if there is a shoulder problem, it may mean they cannot reach up to change a light bulb, towel-dry themselves after a bath, lift a cup and so on. It is important to establish this because, as the treatments progress over a period of weeks, it provides a marker as to how much they are improving; people very quickly forget pain when it is gone. I also ask clients to describe their pain to me, but this is often where they find that they do not have the vocabulary, so I might offer "stitching," "tearing," "dull'," "stabbing," "sharp," "throbbing," "deep," "moving," "vulnerable," and so on. This gives me clues about how I will treat the area, but more importantly, it encourages the client to focus internally, increasing their interoceptive awareness.

As your skills develop over time, in practice you become better able to figure out which path to take as the questioning unfolds in any one session. Without experience, knowledge, and insight, the focus can easily be lost and the answers stop leading to more questions, while also not providing any useful information.

The following are some other questions you might like to ask, leading to conversations around the treatment itself. To lend you both confidence in the treatment, and to give the recipient autonomy, it is important to ask:

- Does the area feel weak and vulnerable?

- Are you nervous about this area being touched?

- Is it sore to the touch?

You can also enquire:

- Do you feel it needs me to get in there and work it really hard?

- Would it feel good to you if I went in slowly?

- Does the pain or restriction feel deep or superficial?

These questions really help the receiver to have a deeper awareness of themselves and to take notice of their body in a way they may not have done before.

I often say this: "I invite you to notice the difference between discomfort and exquisite pain. I will work to a deep level but it should always feel on the right side of pain; it should feel as if it is hitting the spot and is necessary. Please do speak up if it is too much or not enough." This is both helpful for you as the practitioner in judging the efficacy of your treatment, and empowering for the recipient, ensuring that they receive what they need.

Side note: Please remember that even when you have asked a client to speak up, they may well not do so. Check in with them now and again, especially if you see them flinch or feel them tense up. It is vitally important to apply the exact right level of pressure and to make sure the treatment is as perfect as you can make it.

18

How to Touch: A Therapeutic Approach

I often tell the following two stories just to highlight how important it is to study and practice this particular healing art without hurting someone. The nature of Thai yoga massage is that it often, but not always, involves deep work, movement, and stretching, any of which can cause injury if they are not carried out with care and precision.

Many years ago, I had a friend who was training in Thai massage with another teacher. She misheard him say "When working on the sternum, you should *not* use body weight." She thought he had told her to *use* her body weight. So when she came to work on this area on my body, she leaned her whole body weight on to her hand, which was placed on my sternum. We both heard the crack and I felt a soaring pain. It took many months for me to feel better and these days it is still a psychologically vulnerable area, despite the physical body having long since healed. This is a very good lesson to learn from, and when I tell it to my students they all gasp in horror. I know they will not repeat the mistake and will keep in their minds the potential to cause harm easily if not carrying out the work with care and attention. The nature of Thai massage is that it is carried out with leaning pressure, so the practitioner must have an acute awareness of their weight.

Earth element is solid and offers resistance when pushed against, yet my sternum broke when it took the force of my friend's hand. But in doing so, it saved me from much more serious harm, as my lungs and other organs were protected.

The second injury happened not long after, when I had a tendon snapped by a student I was teaching. He was working on my hand and pushed my finger backwards without supporting it. He did not feel for a natural point of resistance, or work with a careful speed to establish the therapeutic limit when applying the stretch to my hand. It happened so suddenly, before I had a chance to guide him. I had to work for weeks one-handed. Despite this, my tendon, an Earth element body part, healed and regenerated with no lasting damage done.

The lesson to learn from these examples is to work with concentration, asking for lots of feedback while practicing. If you are unsure about something, then leave it out until you can check with your teacher.

Chapter 18

There are countless minutiae involved in learning how to touch, some of which are not easy to appreciate from a book and which really need the presence of a teacher to facilitate. However, spending time experimenting safely with these suggestions with a partner should lead you to deeper reflection on the therapeutic experience of touching a body. Many of the following suggestions come from words I frequently speak to students in class.

Thai massage is Buddhist medicine. It requires the practitioner to be very present and focused in the here and now. Thai massage often involves very deep and specific work, which can be dangerous if it is not performed correctly. To be able to work effectively and safely, your eyes must be kept open at all times.

Everything you do in Thai bodywork, every tool you bring out of your toolkit, should be called on for good reason. Be clear about what you are working on (which layer, area, or direction) and why. This way, you do not waste time working on an area that does not need it, or one that you have already addressed. Map out in your mind what you are aiming to achieve. This means that your work will achieve very definite and effective results, and will also be time-efficient. Clients always prefer bodywork that is tailored to their needs and concentrated on what can benefit them most, rather than a standard sequence that very quickly ends up being repetitive and boring for both you and them. Sometimes, this means working in one area for the entire allocated time, and mostly it means that the whole body is not addressed in one session. If you are working thoroughly and therapeutically, there will not be time for everywhere to be worked on, even if two hours are available. Despite this way of working being more concentrated and less general, it is as relaxing and beneficial for the person as a whole-body massage – in fact, more so. Having a treatment that works into the painful area enough for it not to hurt anymore is very relaxing and has lasting effects.

The element system is complex and requires years of study and use to really put into practice, but even with a basic understanding it can guide some treatment choices, tailoring them to the individual.

Palpation

One of the first things I do when I have finished a consultation and the recipient is ready for treatment is to lay my hands on them. Palming (**palpation**) is a time for sensing the quality of soft tissue, muscle, and fascia, and to gain insight into what is going on in that particular area, how bound up it may be. It is a time to feel for quality and texture, and to be aware of sore and tender places.

Palpation is also an important initial touch input that can relax the recipient and create a connection with them; it expresses your confidence of touch. While palpating, I often talk with the client to see how they feel the area, as this encourages their participation in the treatment and puts their attention on themselves, awakening a deeper internal awareness. During this time, they may also comment on or remember a trauma to an area, or mention something about their body that they had forgotten during the consultation. Palpation should be gentle; it is a time to cultivate a very sensitive awareness of what you can feel in the recipient's body. Because of this, it is important not to poke and prod with the fingers but to use your hand sensitively, holding it relaxed and flat.

The "palming" technique, whereby the palm is used to walk up and down an area, is purely a palpatory one. It works well if it is performed skillfully. A sudden application of pressure to the receiver's body will create resistance to that touch. This happens when the hand lifts too far away from the body before moving to the next place to palpate. When some contact is maintained, the hand does not land down on the body, and it is not a sudden or shocking type of touch. A sudden touch feels like an unwelcome surprise each time it creates contact and prevents the receiver from enjoying it. There is a harder quality to the hand when palming like this. Use alternate hand pressure to palpate the area and really be connected to the information you receive from their body.

Other palpatory techniques may involve a gentle stroke, made with all the fingers across an area, feeling very sensitively for changes in heat or searching for bound-up fibers in an area of pain or a site where a problem may arise.

Side note: Something I see frequently in class when teaching is students poking and prodding to locate something specific. It is worth noting here that this is not helpful for the practitioner and it is certainly not pleasant for the recipient. It cannot teach you anything about a structure because the receiver will tense up, contracting the very muscle or area from which you were hoping to get information.

The "Bite" or "End-feel" (Stretching and Pressure)

A common misconception about Thai massage is that it is *always* very deep, and that a large percentage of the treatment is made up of *many* dynamic and *frequently* intense stretches that often verge on the kind of painful approach that means you need to bite on a rag to bear it: the kind of touch where the boundary between pleasure and pain is debatable.

I have found that people respond best to treatment when the pressure or "stretching" is within a comfortable, albeit strong and deep, range, rather than being pushed too far beyond what feels good. There is a fine line between real pain and exquisite pain, and the difference is often a minuscule amount. Finding this balance requires the practitioner to maintain a strong focus at all times: there is no room for error because you can easily injure someone.

Side note: If you see the recipient writhing from your touch, this is an unconscious response as their body tries to escape, so this is a time to reduce the pressure and adjust to their needs. If their central nervous system is ready for action, you are stimulating a fight or flight response, the opposite of the resting and repairing parasympathetic nervous system response.

There are times when the tension clients experience in their body is so acute that it seems that the only way to release it is with prolonged forced pressure or intensification of a stretch. This may feel good in the moment, but in the long run it does not encourage the body to heal itself. When a client is already in pain, they do not need more pain to make them better. For a nervous system that is in overdrive, a painful touch is not going to be healing. The tissues need to be treated with intelligence and curiosity, exploring the area layer by layer to coax movement into it, applying friction or compressions that encourage the body's healing response. There is a big difference between forced hard pressure and a compression that leans into the area, slowly sinking in with skill and without force. When pressure is applied this way, it is easy to find the "bite" or "limit." The "bite" can be extended further, with the right kind of touch and skillful awareness of the response of the tissue.

When it comes to "stretching," it is good to understand that there is a lot of elastic potential in the body. However, using another analogy, imagine you are holding a pair of tights and you stretch them this way; eventually, they will lose elasticity. Stretching is applied to work on the tissue layer (and the Sên). Tight muscles need to be encouraged to stretch and move, but tense muscles must be worked on with techniques that release the tension; they do not generally need stretching more. The goal is to encourage tissues to have fluidity, juiciness, and pliability, and for the Sên to be unrestricted by bound-up tissue so they can function correctly. Ease is felt when there is good, healthy movement in a fluid body. It might be that a smaller fascial stretch that targets tiny muscle fibers facilitates this, while the health of the body's fascial matrix and elastic potential is maintained.

Direct Attention

Focus your attention on what is happening between your body and the recipient's. Information is constantly going back and forth between both of you. Be aware of your touch input, but at the same time your focus must be on what information you feel coming from the recipient's body. There is a two-way communication system at work. If you proceed with this type of concentrated touch, it refines the practice, giving touch and information, receiving information through touch.

Using Earth

We use the Earth of our body to massage the Earth of someone else's body. What this means is that our skin, soft tissue, bones, fascia, central nervous system, and so on are all involved in carrying out a massage. The same Earth body parts of the recipient are being massaged. It is the hardness of our forearm, skin, muscle, fascia, and bone that can roll over the skin, muscles, fascia, and bone of the receiver's foot or shoulder.

Melting Touch

Side note: These names are not traditional but are used to help you form a sense of their quality.

Superficial fascia is a whole-body, sponge-like coating that varies in depth, from thick to thin. It is a second-layer Earth body part but has a high content of Water element; hence it likes to be squeezed, twisted, and rolled on, just like a sponge. The superficial fascia is an intelligent tissue full of blood vessels and nerve endings. It is an intelligent antenna. Your hand, elbow, knee, or foot can melt into the tissue layer of the client's body by slowing down the application of touch. At a reduced speed, there is a completely different and very concentrated, deep but soothing application of touch.

Often, I observe a student pressing into the receiver's body. It is not exactly brute strength that I am witnessing, but they are trying really hard to provide deep pressure and, in doing so, there is a hard, Earthy element to their touch, which does not feel so good. When I suggest that they use a melting touch, everything changes. The student relaxes, their whole body softens, and the receiver always comments that it is a much more pleasurable and therapeutic experience.

The Listening Hand

It is a skill to be able to listen through touch to the subtle qualities of the body. This can be achieved through practicing and developing a strong level of connection and awareness. This delicate, refined approach can add to the healing experience for the client.

The "listening hand" is really a very attentive level of skilled touch, as if the hands have special X-ray capabilities that heighten the senses, almost reading the body.

What is the body asking for? Learn to listen and be sensitive to the condition and texture of each layer of the body. For some people, this ability may be acquired very naturally and quickly, while others will need to allow time to develop this aspect. I suggest starting with sensing through a couple of layers of fabric, and then, as your confidence grows, as you develop your ability to "listen," you can add more and more layers of fabric and continue to explore your sensitivity. This can also be used to build awareness for working with

pulse diagnosis and feeling the subtle changes in Wind Gate work.

Sequencing

When massaging a limb using general, non-specific compressions to warm up an area, there is a sequence of 1–2–3–2–1, which relates to the repetition of hand-positioning that is required to perform them. Following this sequence most of the time means that the receiver will subconsciously be aware of a reassuring set pattern, which is helpful in encouraging their body and mind to go into a deeper relaxed state. Sequencing like this adds up to five compressions. The practitioner could also make the sequence longer (1–2–3–2–1–2–3–2–1), the compressions adding up to nine. Usually, the repetitions will be odd numbers. This sequencing works well for repetitive thumbing of the channels. It means that you avoid having tiny spaces between thumb placements, which would tire the thumbs from overuse.

There is a balanced number of compressions or repetition of touch that aids relaxation or effects most change. Too few is not effective. It is therefore important for the practitioner to know why each repetition is necessary. If there are not enough, it leaves the receiver feeling deprived; if there are more than is needed and the work is done, the receiver may feel restless as they are ready for you to move on.

The number of repetitions depends on the area and layer that are being worked. This cannot be planned for in advance and is another example of why the practitioner must "listen" with the hands and be focused in the present moment.

Effective Stretching

To fine-tune how to perfect a stretch or a compression with stretch, it is important not to overwork. The stretch is often repeated as needed, with each repeat being taken slightly further. A common mistake is for the practitioner to overwork. In such an instance, the stretch looks too bouncy, the receiver experiences the techniques as uncoordinated or ineffective, and the practitioner is unnecessarily working too hard.

When the receiver is taken into the first of the stretches, the stretch should be released only a small way back before they are taken into the second movement. The stretch is then released a small way back again, before moving into the next one. By releasing a stretch in this way only, it is much less work for the practitioner and keeps the attention focused on the technique or stretch being applied. Thus, the move feels much more effective and controlled. This should be repeated until you have achieved what you wanted to and there has been a change.

Confident Touch

You need to move the recipient's body from one position to another and carry out techniques with confidence. It feels much better if you are definite and this ensures that the recipient relaxes more, being assured of your skill and proficiency. Be decisive in how you shift the receiver into a new position, moving their body definitely rather than tentatively, as this enables deeper relaxation. You can always use a transition from one move to another that keeps the fluid element of the session intact (see more in Chapter 19).

The Hard or Soft Tool

If the hand is used with fingers straight, the pressure is harder and stronger than with fingers curled. Similarly, when using the forearm, a clenched fist will harden the tissue around the ulna, which will give a deeper pressure than if the fist is relaxed (Fig. 18.1).

Fine-tuning

There are many small details that make a technique accurate. It really takes focus, reflection, and practice, as sometimes even changing a

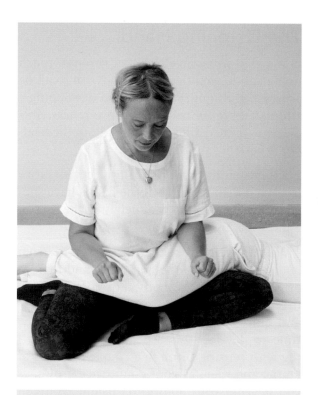

Fig. 18.1
Clenched fists create harder pressure.

position by just a few millimeters makes a vast difference to its efficacy. It is important for the arm to be sitting comfortably in the shoulder joint, so that its trajectory, when being taking into the overhead stretch, is effective. A slight arc is needed for it to be correct.

Angles

Angles of 45 or 90 degrees are generally the correct positions for the recipient's limbs to be massaged or stretched. The angle of a practitioner's hand, thumb, or arm when working is also important for the application to be easily effective.

Speed

Speed is important and will need to be adjusted for each person. The more you understand about core element constitution (CEC; see Chapter 5), the easier it will be to adapt your speed to meet the frequency (or needs) of the individual. For example, when working with someone who is CEC Water and who has agitated Water, they will have much more Watery tissue than usual. The speed you work at to help set the fluids moving will need to be faster than if you were working on a Fiery CEC person (who generally needs longer holds to calm the Fire). You need to be careful that the faster pace for the Watery person still attains the correct depth of pressure. Working at a faster pace does not mean missing the "bite." If you are working on a Windy CEC, the speed must not aggravate their Winds by being too fast or too slow. You need to be really sensitive to their response so that you make it perfect for them, working with a balanced speed.

19 Body Mechanics

When I first started out as a Thai massage practitioner, it was the stretches that I enjoyed giving most. Nowadays, despite giving far fewer stretches in treatments, there is something very fulfilling about knowing how to move someone around with ease, grace, and confidence. To work effectively, you must know how to use your body so that you do not tire or injure yourself.

How you move your body and how smoothly you move around during a session have an impact on the flow of the whole massage and on how much confidence the recipient feels in the practitioner. Here we look at correct body mechanics, what is good movement, and how you know when it is not.

The accurate use of body weight to provide and adapt pressure is vital to ensure safe practice for the practitioner's body, as well as providing an effective experience for the recipient.

The efficient movement of the practitioner's body ensures that the receiver's body is also moved smoothly: the two are interlinked. Inefficient movement, where there is tension or hard work, drains the practitioner so that muscles are overused and tiredness sets in. This is not something that can be maintained over years and could cause long-term injury to the practitioner.

The strength of the massage is often misleading to the receiver, who is mostly lying with eyes closed in the session. It may seem as if the practitioner is working very hard, applying compressions and moving the limbs into various positions, whereas when the practitioner is skilled they will be feeling relaxed, using their body to lean into the work effortlessly (Fig. 19.1).

Gravity is a key factor in giving a Thai massage. The practitioner works with a neutral spine and is most often positioned directly above, or at a 45-degree angle to, the receiver's body. The use of gravity, combined with the practitioner working smart, not hard, by moving into the work, ensures minimum effort.

On a floor mat there is versatility so that working positions can be adapted to always be comfortable, whether standing, kneeling, side-sitting, or lunging. The fundamental rule of thumb is to place a hand, knee, or foot on to the recipient's body and lean *into* it using the natural pull of gravity, which avoids there being any need for strength or hard work.

Chapter 19

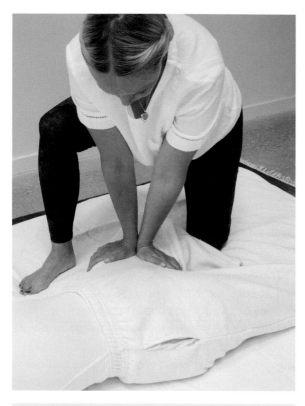

Fig. 19.1
The practitioner keeps the arms straight and leans into the work while letting the shoulders travel beyond the wrists to give effortless, intensified bodywork.

Side note: Thai Massage does not have to be performed on a floor mat. It can be given on a chair, massage table, or low massage bed. It is not what the massage is done on that defines it as Thai massage, but more specifically the approach of the practitioner and the perspective of Thai medical theory.

The majority of techniques will be carried out with the practitioner facing the receiver so that they can watch the responses and see the visual reactions. This is often a helpful way to gauge their limitations. Most rules (for example, always lean into a move) are not set in stone, as there are definitely times when facing away or leaning back is a more efficient use of body mechanics. Knowing when, how, and why something needs one approach and not another comes with practice on many different bodies and guidance from a teacher.

Transfer of Weight

Dancers understand about transfer of weight, and it is significant for a Thai practitioner to recognize this as a way to move and use the body. It refers to the placement and alteration of body weight and your center of gravity. When you lean on to a foot, hand, or knee, you are transferring weight to that area. Each time you slide your working foot or hand to the next place on the receiver's body, the weight is transferred to the non-working foot or hand.

There are many areas of the body that can be used in Thai massage, and at any one time there could be two or more points of contact to carry out a technique effectively.

In the example shown in Figure 19.2, we can see that the hands are holding the receiver's foot. The practitioner is standing on one leg and the other foot is against the receiver's sacrum, stabilizing it in position. The practitioner must carefully transfer weight on to the active foot to lean on to the body. To accomplish this with skill, there must be a precise transfer of weight to ensure that there is not too much pressure applied but that it is enough to be effective. The working foot is active but

This balanced mid point will be different, depending on whether the recipient is heavier or lighter than you. The practitioner needs to be able to adjust to this during each lift by staying rooted to the floor and maintaining concentration (Fig. 19.3).

Thai massage is simple in many ways, yet conversely complex in others. Many aspects need to be combined together. Thai massage takes practice and perseverance, and a depth of understanding that comes from dedication to the practice, on-going study, and reflection.

It is worth noting that, as you first practice, you will be using your body in new ways and this can lead to temporary muscular soreness, especially when you go over a section or particular technique many times as you try to perfect or fine-tune it.

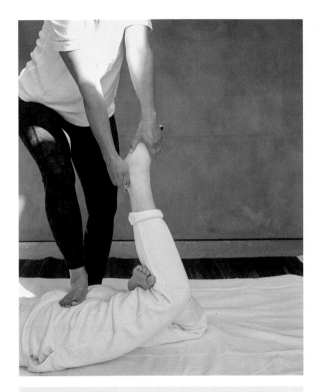

Fig. 19.2
Fixing the sacrum and lifting the leg to the correct height whilst maintaining a mid point of distributed weight.

the practitioner's standing leg will be taking the majority of the weight.

Counterbalancing during Lifts

There are some lifts that involve the practitioner using the weight of the recipient's body to make the move effective and stable. At these times, the practitioner must use that weight properly. Navigate the weight of both bodies to find the center of balance between you, which is the mid point. Finding this makes the move easy and safe to give and effective to receive.

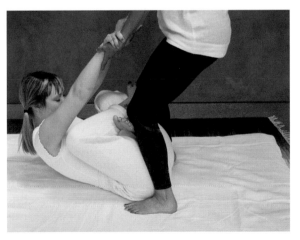

Fig. 19.3
The weight of the recipient's body counterbalances the lift, which then allows the practitioner to tilt their own pelvis anteriorly and have a small back bend, which increases the lift.

Chapter 19

Different Strokes for Different Folks

Each client you work on will be different to the next. You will need to learn to adjust the angles of your working postures to the size of each body. The angle and use of your body in relation to theirs directly impacts on the efficacy of the moves. They will vary according to the size, shape, weight, length, and breadth of the individual.

Recommendations for Appropriate Body Mechanics

General

Make sure that you are comfortable and relaxed at all times. If you are tense or uncomfortable, you will tire very easily and will not benefit from the experience yourself. Your discomfort will be picked up on by the receiver, who will also enjoy the experience less. If you cannot find a way of being comfortable when trying to carry out a particular move, adjust how you perform it. Sometimes, a tiny adjustment makes a massive difference.

Technique is much more important than strength. We need to use our bones to lift, rather than muscles that tire easily. You can see that in Figure 9.3. The weight of the recipient is being taken by the practitioner's legs, not their back. *Always* lift with your legs.

Keep your limbs straight (but not locked). For example, an arm that is bent at the elbow will lose its strength. Any bend in a joint will make the practitioner use muscle strength and they will be working hard, but not smart. It also makes the work much less effective.

When using your hands and thumbs, make sure that the joints of your arm are stacked in line – shoulder over elbow over wrist.

Keep your spine aligned in neutral and your shoulders relaxed. Maintaining your own alignment during a session ensures comfort and ease of movement, while avoiding straining the body or using too much strength.

In general, check that your neck and spine are straight and in line with each other, and that you are not tilting the head or flexing the neck. However, there are times when it is necessary to flex the neck, so just be aware that you are not working in this way unnecessarily.

Ensure that you work with your pelvis neither anteriorly nor posteriorly tilted, as this could weaken the lumbar spine and cause injury.

Keep yourself rooted to the ground and balanced, which will ensure that you do not fall on to the recipient. Making sure that your feet are fully in contact with the floor means that you are working from a stable position (Fig. 19.4).

Ensure that you move your body to the correct place to be certain that you are not over-reaching or straining. In doing this, you will apply an equal and direct amount of pressure to the area you are working on and will keep your body aligned and comfortable.

Never balance on both of your knees at the same time when applying pressure (that is, make sure you keep a foot on the floor), to maintain a stable position.

When pulling or pressing, keep your arms straight but not rigid; do not lock the elbows, as this will put strain on the joint (Fig. 19.5).

The ideal foot position is to have the toes tucked (not flat). In this way, they can be used

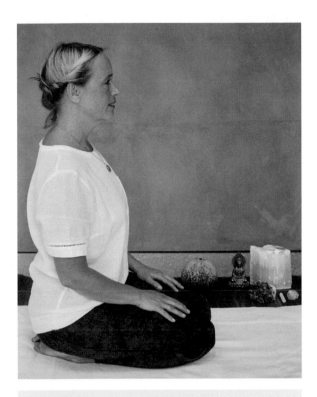

Fig. 19.4
Flattened feet for a lower working position.

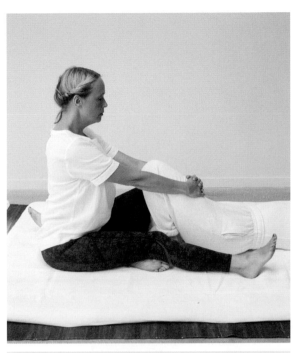

Fig. 19.5
Forearms and hands grip the upper leg and the practitioner leans back to apply this stretch for the hip flexors and sacrum

to take energy from the ground. The plantar fascia of the foot has tensile strength, and this works with the ground like a spring from which all movements can be made (Fig. 19.6). This is not an absolute rule – there are times when flat feet are better, as the working position is then closer to the ground.

Lifts

Lift with your legs not your back, keeping your knees bent as you lift (Fig. 19.7).

Let most of the weight of the receiver go into your legs as you lift.

Keep your arms straight, unless you want to intensify the stretch at the end of it by bending your elbows to pull more.

Use the breath if the recipient is holding on; this directs their focus to something else.

If working with the breath, you can synchronize your breath with theirs by doing opposite breathing – as you lift, they breathe in and you breathe out. As you release, they breathe out and you breathe in.

To increase a lift, tilt your pelvis anteriorly and look up.

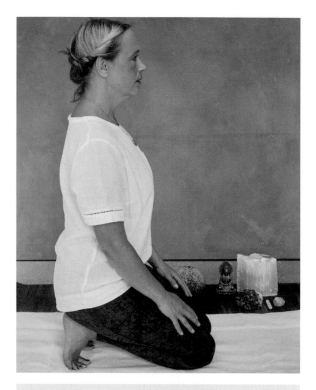

Fig. 19.6
The plantar fascia is spring-loaded and gives energy to a stable working position.

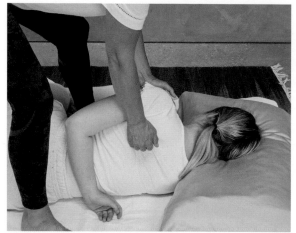

Fig. 19.7
Lift with bent knees to ensure correct body mechanics. The weight goes into the practitioner's legs, not back.

Compressions with Hands

When you are leaning on to your palms, your arms should be straight but not locked; a micro-bend is all that needed.

Position your body so that you can lean in, but from a distance, as compressions will be deeper this way. Having space to move into the work enables deeper pressure if it is needed.

Allow your shoulders to go beyond your wrists for effective and deeper compressions that also stretch fascia.

Keep your whole hand (fingers included) in contact with the receiver's body; make sure it is relaxed for softer pressure, but keep your fingers straight for harder pressure.

If you are using thumbing technique, you can apply counterpressure with your fingers or keep your fingers active.

If you are working one-handed, you can place one hand on top of the other or your non-working hand can grasp the forearm of your working hand; this helps keep the connection and strength of touch, and is a traditional way to work.

Compressions with Feet

Feet are used in Thailand only when they are the best tool for the job, never for show. They are seen as dirty or unclean in Thai culture.

In general, use the insteps or balls of your feet on the area you are massaging.

If you are using toes, make sure you feel comfortable and stable.

If you are using one foot to work with when standing, ensure you have good balance or something to hold on to.

Use and adjust body weight for effective leaning.

Feet provide broad pressure.

If you are standing, remember that you will be using your whole body weight until you transfer weight to the other foot.

Blading with the foot gives very deep pressure. The practitioner uses the outside edge of the foot when blading (see Chapter 20).

The calcaneus can be used to apply heel compressions in a standing or seated position. When standing, the practitioner has the benefit of gravity and whole body weight (Fig. 19.8); when seated, the calcaneus is often used to slowly "melt" into the tissue of the upper body. When used around the gluteal muscles, its focus is to create space away from the sacrum (Fig. 19.9).

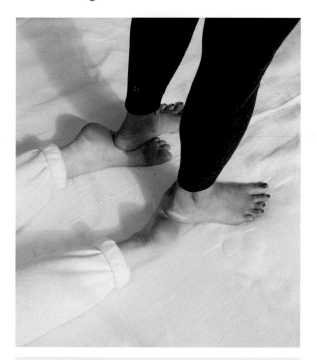

Fig. 19.8
Using the calcaneus as a massage tool on the plantar fascia.

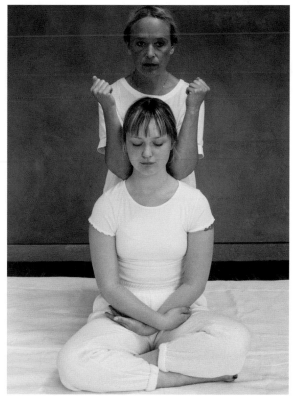

Fig. 19.9
Precise point work with elbows.

151

Compressions with Elbows

Elbows have three bones that can be used for massage: the olecranon and the medial and lateral epicondyles. Make sure you know which one you are using by keeping a visual focus until you have developed strong neural pathways of awareness to this area.

Be aware that your elbow is particularly pointed and applies deep, focused, or intense pressure, so work with care (Fig. 19.10).

Use body weight to lean into the area you are working on.

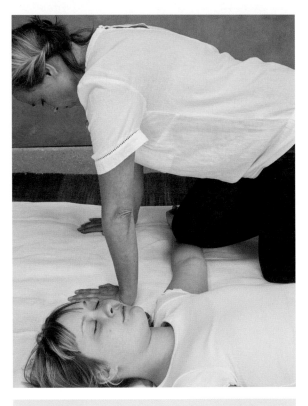

Fig. 19.10
The patellar tendon is used to apply pressure.

Compressions with Knees

Knees provide a broad and very deep pressure.

It is easy to misjudge how much pressure is being applied, as knees do not know their own strength.

Make sure you maintain balance by transferring weight.

Be aware of your body weight.

Transfer your weight to your non-working leg to adapt pressure.

Use the lower/flat part of the patella (patellar tendon), not the patella itself (Fig. 19.11).

Correct Alignment of the Receiver

Throughout the session, the recipient will become increasingly relaxed. Sometimes, this

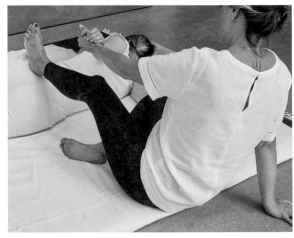

Fig. 19.11
Using the calcaneus on the piriformis and gluteus muscles.

means that their body becomes quite floppy. At other times, you may have performed stretches on one side of the body, and before you move on to the other side you might notice the receiver is no longer angled correctly. In these situations, to make the session go smoothly and to ensure that you are able to continue massaging effectively, you may need to realign the receiver. Try to do this decisively with minimum disruption. You may also be able to find seamless ways to move them into alignment by performing transitions.

Transitions

The ability of the Thai practitioner to move the receiver's body from one technique to the next without disrupting the flow is key to perfecting the stretching part of the massage. These movements between moves are what I call transitions. A transition often needs as much practice as any other technique but it is these finer details that take the massage to another level. The main stipulation for any of the transitions is that they allow one stretch to flow to the next. There are no rules about how transitions are given; the important aspect is to make it seem a natural and simple way to progress from one move to the next. Once you start to be familiar with the body and a client's individual range of motion, it is possible to be really creative when transitioning between moves. Each transition then becomes part of the healing, in that it incites the recipient to "let go" of their own motor control. A transition can include stretches, and the passive movement of a limb into position using the natural range of the joint articulation. A transition is the fluid journey from one move to another.

Gravity

Gravity is used within Thai massage to give pressure by leaning down. The practitioner can also use the weight of the receiver's body and gravity to work from underneath their body. For example, the knee might be underneath the gluteal region to apply pressure to it (Fig. 19.12).

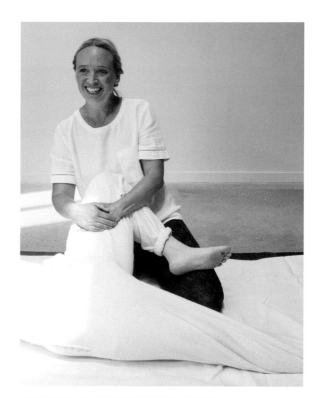

Fig. 19.12
The therapist's knee is placed under the recipient's body and their weight is used to intensify the compression. Hands hold the leg and create an additional stretch of the adductor.

Working Postures

- *Low, sitting on the heels* – sit on your heels with your feet flat against the floor. Knees can be open or closed.

- *Mid-height, sitting on the heels* – sit on your heels, with your feet flexed and toes against the floor. Knees can be open or closed.

- *High-kneeling* – come up on to your knees; feet can be flat or tucked under, and knees should be hip-width apart (Fig. 19.13).

- *Crawling* – kneel on all fours with knees under your hips and wrists below the shoulders. Keep your back flat. Arms are straight but without locking the elbows.

- *Proposal pose* – place one foot flat on the floor in front of you and kneel on the other leg (Fig. 19.14).

- *Extended proposal pose* – place one foot flat on the floor further in front of you. Kneel on the other leg.

- *Side lunge* – kneel in proposal pose with one leg on the floor and bring the other leg out to your side, keeping your foot flat on the floor.

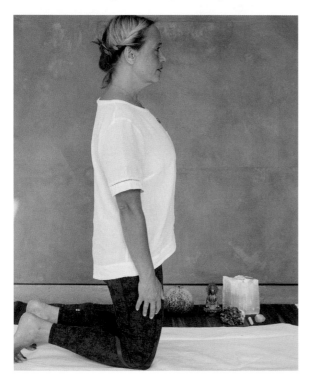

Fig. 19.13
The high-kneeling position is used when the recipient is seated and for some pulling techniques.

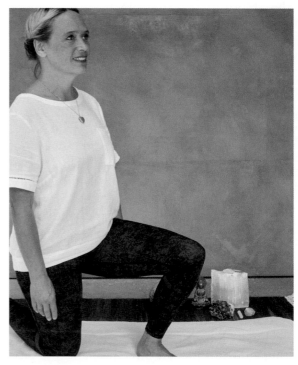

Fig. 19.14
Proposal pose is a working position that allows easy movement for the practitioner.

- *Side-sitting* – sit with your bottom on the floor and both legs bent to one side of you.

- *Wide knee squatting* – place both feet on the floor. Knees can be wide or hip-width apart. Let your bottom travel towards your heels. You may be more comfortable being on the balls of your feet rather than having flat feet.

- *One foot squat* – sit on one heel with toes flexed and your knee against the floor. Place your other foot flat on the floor (Fig. 19.15).

- *Full squat* – place both feet on the floor with knees apart and your hips low to the ground.

- *Side squat* – sit on your heel with toes flexed. Let your other leg go out to the side of you, keep your foot flat on the floor.

- *Seated four-leg* – sit on your bottom with one leg in front of you and the other foot close to the pelvis.

- *Standing lunge* – take a big step forwards, placing your foot on the floor directly in front of you. Bend your knee. Straighten your other leg behind you.

- *Stepping* – stand with feet hip-width apart. Take a step forwards and straighten the back leg. Bend the knee of your working leg. Transfer weight as necessary (Fig. 19.16).

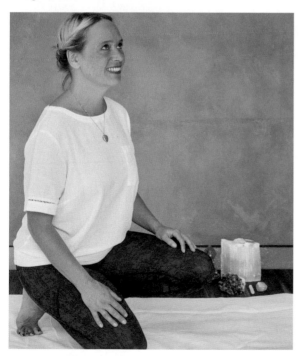

Fig. 19.15
A one-foot squat provides the ability for movement in a low position.

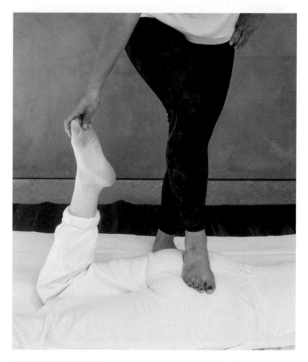

Fig. 19.16
Stepping on to the body with one foot.

Breath

The breath is the bridge between the subtle and gross Winds.

Breath *is* life-giving movement. The rhythm of the breath can be very telling. Is the recipient's breathing tense, holding, steady, staggered, labored, fast, shallow, deep, full? Does it ebb and flow like the tide, expand and contract the ribcage and diaphragm to massage the belly and organs?

The physiological effects of the breath are far-reaching. The whole body, from foot to stomach to scalp, breathes with the lungs as the movement of the breath unifies the whole. The steady rhythm of the heart gently communicates its beat to the lungs, stimulating them over and over – up to 20,000 times a day; their intimate relationship depends on it. The liver, stomach, diaphragm, and beyond feel the reverberations of this natural phenomenon. Oxygenated blood, its content dependent on

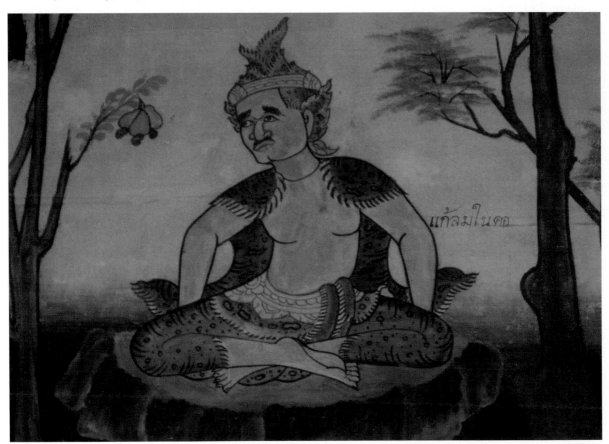

Fig. 19.17
Reusi Dat Ton posture. With kind permission of David Wells.

the quality of the breath, is carried around the body, nourishing muscles and fascia as they, too, move. The expansion and contraction of each breath massage vessels, arteries, neural offshoots. A breath can help let go of the old and can breathe in new life. Your first and last breaths complete the cycle of your life.

> "Your lungs, those fluttering butterfly wings of your heart, shape your other organs as well, living as they do in the tidal ebb and flow of your breath waves lapping at those visceral shores."
>
> Gil Hedley, personal communication, 2016

While giving a Thai massage, the practitioner will need to keep relaxed breathing. If the practitioner holds their breath, it creates tension in their own body, disrupting the ease of the session for both participants.

When the practitioner is performing specific techniques, asking clients to focus on their breathing is a helpful tool to aid relaxation, encourage letting go, and provide an internal focal point. In Thai massage, an inhalation is taken as the pressure, stretch, or lift is applied, and as the recipient releases their breath the technique is released. This is something that many people struggle to come to grips with, as they are so firmly rooted in the more modern, Yogic way of breathing out on the exertion. I always suggest that people try it many times as they practice Thai massage, both giving and receiving it, so this breathing technique can be fully experienced. It is powerful to release the breath as the deep pressure or stretch is released because everything can let go at once. This way of breathing is an ancient technique that was used by the Reusi in Reusi Dat Ton (Thai yoga; Fig. 19.17).

If you are trying to perform a technique and the receiver is holding on or tense, this will prevent the technique being performed accurately or effectively. If the receiver is not finding it easy to allow you to move their body into a posture, they are not yet relaxed. Using breathing as a focus is extremely helpful, partly as a distraction technique.

Side note: Practitioners should carry out *opposite* breathing to the recipient (in on the exertion, out when releasing the technique). They should take care not to make a really big deal about their breathing pattern. I say this because there have been many times when I have seen a practitioner being so focused on their own breath that it is unnecessarily loud and dramatic.

Breath focus can be used, but is not something that is required continuously.

There are times when your client will lie down on the mat, and you will notice that their breath is not relaxed or is very shallow. This meditation is a wonderful way to get them connected to themselves and begin to relax.

A Breathing Meditation

This meditation is to encourage the recipient to have a deeper internal focus, to notice details about themselves which they may not have been previously aware of, and to have gratitude for their life and body in a very simple way. Give these instructions and ask these questions quietly so they can reflect within themselves:

- Close your eyes and take your attention to your breath.

- Notice that you *are* breathing.

- Feel this breath and notice that it signifies how alive you are.

- Appreciate your breath, no matter the pace, ease, or fullness.

- Ask yourself where your breath is.

- Do you feel it in your chest, belly, mouth, or nose?

- Feel it at the front of your body, that rising and falling.

- Bring awareness to the breath at the back of your body, expanding/contracting.

- Do you feel a sense of holding on anywhere?

- Are there areas that you do not feel connected to?

- Breathe into yourself; direct your breath where it needs to go.

- Let the rhythm of your breath massage you there.

- Let the waves from your heart flutter the wings of your lungs as they massage you free of charge.

- Observe every part of you as you breathe.

- Notice every part of you working together and as one.

- Connect your breath to your heart and send this energy to any area of your body that needs love.

Intimacy, Space, and Culture

There is a lot of physical closeness in Thai massage, which makes it unique. Many parts of the body are used, requiring the practitioner to carry out the massage with increased whole-body awareness (Fig. 19.18). There is a fine line

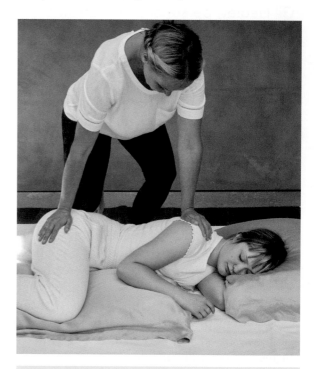

Fig. 19.18
The practitioner must work with high levels of whole-body concentration.

between keeping close contact that is comfortable and professional, and physical closeness that is too much so that the receiver feels their privacy has been invaded.

Throughout the massage, there will be times when there could be many points of physical contact between both people. Some points of contact may be incidental and additional to the move. These often arise when the contact makes things easier on the practitioner's body or provides stability to the technique. It increases the level of physical connection and makes it more comfortable for both participants. An example of this is when the massage is being performed predominantly with the arms to one area of their body, but there may also be contact with the practitioner's legs and abdomen (Fig. 19.19). This adds depth to the whole-body approach and gives a distinctive experience of close touch. It is also representative of an Eastern approach to the body, as closer physicality is culturally more acceptable than in the West, where we are notoriously conscious of our physical space. This additional contact can be nurturing and liberating.

However, if there is a momentary lack of concentration in this whole-body awareness, then this close touch can easily become inappropriate and could prevent the receiver from trusting that they are safe.

There are times when space is also more appropriate than a "body contact" approach. Understanding what is right for your client and making the decision to give more space need to be constantly considered throughout the session. This will vary, depending on the level of trust you have built up with each client and how familiar they are with touch or bodywork.

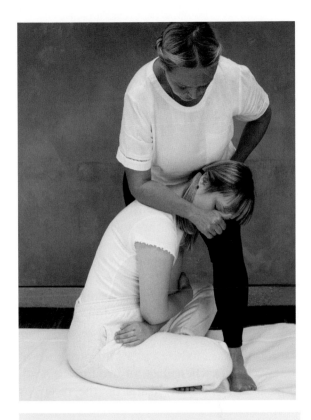

Fig. 19.19
Seated position shoulder work.

There will be areas where close contact is more suitable, and areas where it either does not work, or is too much, or is inappropriate.

Space is often needed between yourself and the receiver to perform a specific technique accurately. It is important to ensure that the practitioner's body does not get in the way, or disrupt fluid movement from one posture to another. It may be that the practitioner's body needs to lean back to lift an area and move it, so that the receiver's body weight is used. In this instance, it is better than leaning forwards, which could strain the practitioner's body and make the move ineffective. An example would be when the practitioner steps on to the hamstrings. The practitioner needs to ensure correct placement of the non-working foot so that when weight is transferred to the working foot it is most effective. The space/distance between the recipient's body and the non-working foot is what aids efficacy.

The more the massage is practiced and fine-tuned, the more accurately the practitioner will be able to judge the distance or proximity needed to create the correct balance of intimacy, space, and effectiveness. This adjustment varies, depending on the size and shape of the practitioner and recipient, and judging this comes with practice and verifies the need for a teacher to be present while becoming familiar with so many variations.

It is important to be aware of the proximity of the two bodies when working around the head. How the giver's body leans on the receiver's body can sometimes be enjoyable, yet at other times can feel awkward and unpleasant. For example, in a seated position, the olecranons are being used bilaterally on the shoulders. As soon as the therapist's hands rest on the head, the body contact becomes too much. The hands on the head feel compressive and unpleasant.

In Thailand, the head is considered a sacred area of the body and this should be

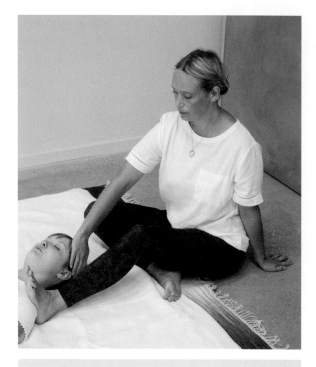

Fig. 19.20
Feet working near the head.

acknowledged during treatment. As much as is feasibly possible, the head area should not have feet pointing at it; nor should the practitioner walk around the head to switch from one side to the other. However, feet can be used near the head as long as they are the best tool for the job (Fig. 19.20).

20 Physical Therapy Toolkit

The mutually supporting and interdependent structures of the body must be acknowledged by the practitioner to ensure efficacy and safety during bodywork that is often deep and intense. Having a perspective of the body as a whole (from superficial to deep, and from the crown of the head to the toes) is the only way that real therapeutic work gets done. Taking this wider view makes for interesting work for the practitioner, and positive treatment outcomes are far greater.

All techniques address more than one layer at a time, and all layers interact with each other. However, the importance of caring for each individual layer of the body before moving to a deeper layer is the only kind of sequence there is in Thai physical therapy. Treating the body this way is like using a map to navigate: there are many routes to follow, but only one direction to travel in.

For example, a client could be experiencing strong pain and limited movement in the right leg. The place to start treatment is likely to be that leg. It could be that the treatment never moves to another area of the body because (after working on the skin, which is generally fairly compliant) it could take some time to penetrate the superficial and deep fascia and

muscle to restore fluid play to them. But until this second layer has a malleable softening texture and feels less painful for the recipient, the next layer should not be addressed.

The muscle and fascia layer is crying out for fluidity and ease of movement, as it easily tends to become bound up, tense, and painful. One of the goals of Thai massage is to introduce movement to these tissues. If and when the second layer is returned to being juicy and malleable, then the third layer of channels and Sên can be worked for deeper physiological efficacy.

In Western anatomy terms, the nerves and vessels are categorized as the neuro-vascular system. Their resemblance to trees, if observed in their entirety, is striking, and for this reason they could be called the nerve and heart trees (see Fig. 10.1). Sên are more encompassing than this, as they also refer to lymph vessels, tendons, ligaments, fallopian tubes, ureters, and all physical pathways of movement in the body that are thin and noodle-shaped.

It is by considering each layer, having patience with the structure of that layer, and being focused and skilled in the choice and application of techniques that the practitioner can bring about a change in the body.

Side note: Sequential Thai massage is often inaccurately described as a "dance" by those who are performing it, the stretches being one continuous flow of movement. However, *therapeutic* Thai massage is very different to this, with the practitioner frequently being still while one area is being deeply compressed or a Wind Gate is being worked. An onlooker might think it is like watching paint dry but the recipient will be receiving very beneficial bodywork.

You need to wait patiently and not move on before the recipient's body is ready. Intense and strong pressure, while painful, can feel extremely healing. The level of "exquisite pain" is right on the edge, but it is sometimes *exactly* what the body is calling out for. There are other times that the body needs something *much* gentler. Pain thresholds vary and are often reflected in the individual's core element constitution (CEC; see Chapter 5) and their functional movement, daily habits, and natural cycles, all of which are influential and affect treatment choices made by the practitioner. When someone is already suffering and in pain, it is wise to be gentle, and a very aware, precise touch is required. The practitioner's hands need to listen.

Fascia does not respond well to sudden and deep pressure, but if the skin and superficial fascia have been worked on and are malleable, then the body is prepared for deeper work into the deep fascia and muscle below. Then, strong touch is not a threat and is often experienced and described as exquisite pain.

Thai bodywork is very relaxing. It can create a sense of calm and restoration, and may be used for many remedial purposes. Some of the techniques may not feel relaxing while they are being performed, as they can be intense and deep, but they feel so good afterwards and have long-lasting effects. Other techniques can be gentle, settling, and restorative, such as the spinal nerve treatment, heart–mind points, or Wind Gate work described in Chapter 22.

Side note: **Access points** are located in specific places in the body, often areas that are busy with Sên or where two muscles cross and layer. These are very sensitive points. The practitioner must work with concentrated attention and subtle touch input. As the points are worked, the practitioner is assessing and waiting for change, carefully observing the client. Access points are different to **release points** (see later in this chapter).

Working therapeutically, the practitioner addresses many aspects of the body to maintain health. These could include: cleaning lymph, moving Winds, balancing the body, treating an injury, realigning the musculoskeletal framework, hydrating and cleansing tissue, balancing elements, increasing circulation and communication, moving stagnation, relieving pain, treating the Sên, calming the mind, and supporting optimum organ function.

Pulse Diagnosis

Pulse reading is a traditional approach to diagnosis. Essentially, the practitioner feels for the rhythm of the Wind moving throughout the body and compares it to the dominant navel pulse of the abdominal aorta.

Fingers are placed initially just below the navel (called the mother pulse). Using three fingers, this pulse is then compared to other pulses at the feet, wrists, and temples. The mother pulse is the strongest pulse due to its close proximity to the abdominal aorta, but it is important to note that if this pulse is weak, abdominal/visceral massage is indicated.

Learning and Applying Massage and Bodywork Techniques

When I first took Thai massage training I learned pressing, thumbing, and stretching techniques, which were put together in a sequence lasting around two hours. Additionally, I was taught a small number of spot-specific release points.

Later, in subsequent training, I learned more stretches, herbal compresses, some rocking techniques, and a scraping technique called **Gua Sha** (which my teacher at that time explained was not Thai but Chinese in origin, and is good at the onset of coughs and colds).

As I became more confident giving treatments, I found that I started to deviate from Thai techniques, sometimes introducing oil and touching the body in ways that I felt were therapeutic but were not grounded in any theory I had been taught. A few years later, I discovered traditional Thai theory and realized that all these massage techniques *were*, in fact, Thai or Lanna. Subsequently, I found out that there are additional tools of the trade, one of which is the application of scraping, which I had previously learned (called Khuut; Fig.

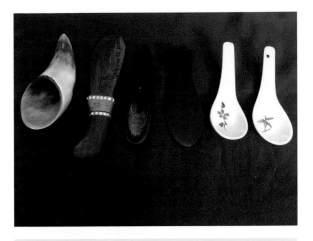

Fig. 20.1
Khuut tools of Thai Bodywork.

20.1), and others such as cupping and herbal compresses (see Chapter 15).

Side note: Khuut is a Lanna medicine technique. Lanna people are from Northern Thailand; they have their own language and do not consider themselves to be Thai. Many techniques found in traditional Thai bodywork *are* Lanna techniques. To this day, the Lanna people have preserved much of the medicine from old times.

Underlying all the techniques of Thai bodywork are Thai medical theory and the five roots. Having some basic knowledge of Thai anatomy and physiology, Buddhism, and the elements of Earth, Water, Fire, Wind, and Space drastically and immediately alters how the practitioner approaches a treatment. For the best treatment outcomes, a deep understanding that comes from years of study, reflection, practice, and observation is required.

Side note: Thai Massage is Buddhist medicine. A practitioner does not have to be Buddhist to practice it, but there are many teachings found in Buddhism that strengthen and deepen the practitioner's understanding of the medicine. They are profoundly interlinked.

Side note: As a point of interest, a Thai massage practitioner traditionally would not learn *any* techniques until Thai medical theory and Buddhism had been studied. Techniques would slowly be introduced to the student when the teacher was happy that the theoretical knowledge, much of it including Buddhist sutras, had been studied. However, it is almost impossible in the modern day to have a relationship with a teacher that means living with or near to them. And so we do the best we can to learn and study and stay curious about all the ways that we can develop our knowledge to best serve our clients' health.

There is a real emphasis on the practitioner being clear about what they are doing and why. It is no good carrying out a technique or protocol if it is not needed. With so many ways to treat the body available, it is important for there to be a good reason to choose each method, which ensures a carefully tailored remedial approach. The theory should lead to a diagnosis of what is needed, and then the techniques should be applied.

There are times when a technique is being carried out and it just feels ineffective. You may know that the technique is being performed accurately and yet it is not working. Usually, I find it is because the technique was not what the recipient needed. If this happens, acknowledge that, despite thinking it would be helpful, it is not, and then move on. Often, it is when your hands begin to work on the body that the information about what is needed becomes clearer: your brain has the knowledge, then your hands feel what to do with that information.

This also flags up the need for deeper understanding of the theory to be able to diagnose properly. The techniques and their application will then be effective.

The Techniques

Thai massage is much more than thumbing, pressing, and stretching. The following section provides examples of other techniques that are available to a traditional therapeutic practitioner. It is not an exhaustive list, as there are many more. Some of these come from the Lanna tradition in the north of Thailand, while others are from central Thailand.

Skin

Rubbing

This is performed with a vigorous and definite touch, rather than a gentle stroking movement. The purpose is to generate heat and warmth, so think in terms of how your mother might have rubbed you dry with a towel after swimming to warm you up. Often, when rubbing is done on bare skin, you can see that it becomes red; this is called **erythema** and is an indication that the vessel trees of the cardiovascular system are reacting and reaching out to the input of touch. Despite rubbing being a technique primarily for the skin layer, it is the perfect way of understanding how, when you touch one aspect of the body, you affect the whole. Rubbing can be done with or without oil, on skin or through clothes. In general, I suggest raw sesame oil (unrefined and organic) when the body needs to be heated a little, or coconut oil for a more cooling substance.

Soft Tissue/Fascia

Forearm rolling

This is a great technique for releasing tension in the second layer. The middle of the forearm should be placed on to the body with the palm facing down, then rolled outwards (away from you) each time. In doing this, the ulna bone massages the body. This technique can be carried out on any area of the body, apart from the head and neck. Clenching your fist will harden the tissue of the arm around the ulna to provide deeper pressure. The movement itself is down into the body with leaning, and the outward roll continues to slide over the underlying fascia (Fig. 20.2).

Squeezing

This is a wonderful way of releasing tense and tight muscles. Generally, the tissue is squeezed between all four fingers and the heel of the hand (the padding of the thumb joint, called the **thenar eminence**), or sometimes the fingers and thumb are used. The superficial fascia is lifted as it is squeezed, which creates space

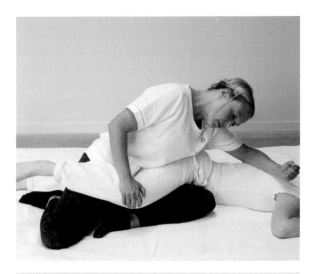

Fig. 20.2
The practitioner uses the weight of the head to deepen this technique.

away from the deeper fascia and encourages it to glide over the filmy fascia in the process. I think of this technique as being one that hydrates the tissues. It is like squeezing a sponge: the fluid is squeezed out and, as the pressure releases, the sponge fills back up with fresh fluids and nutrients. If you concentrate while practicing this repeatedly, you can feel the tissues becoming juicier as they hydrate.

Boyfriend massage

This is a technique that most people know and the name should give a good indication of what it is. It involves using thumbs to press, knead, and generally work into the soft tissue, using fingers as counterpressure. It is a great way to loosen the soft tissue and can also be carried out with balms. A common area for this technique to be used is the shoulders, in seated or prone position.

Chapter 20

Beating (dtee)

There are many ways to beat the body, and the depth of pressure and speed can be adjusted with each beating technique. For it to be effective, it should be performed continuously for *at least* one minute, or it will not effect a change in the tissue. In addition to how good it feels to receive and how beneficial it is for the tissue layer as a dispersing, relaxing, and invigorating technique, each method has a unique sound, which is pleasant to hear. This technique is therapeutic for waking up the nerves and moving deep-rooted stagnation. One thing to remember is that if it sounds like a slap, then it will feel like a slap. You will know when you are doing it right, as there will be an airy, snappy, or hollow sound.

There are several variations:

- With hands in prayer position, the outside edges of the little fingers make contact repeatedly with the recipient's body (Fig. 20.3; this is often named the Thai chop).

- The outside edges of the little fingers can be used alternately to beat the body.

- With loosely clenched fists, the outside edges of the hands are used to beat the body.

- Hands grasp each other (the grip not being too loose or tight) and the backs of the hand (third/fourth/fifth metacarpal area) are used.

- The palms of the hands are held in a slight arc (so they are not flat) and the body is beaten with alternating hands (Fig. 20.4).

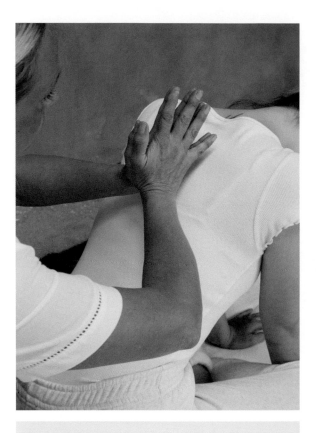

Fig. 20.3
Dtee. This dispersal technique is used for bound-up tissue and can be gentle or strong. Either way, it produces a therapeutic sound.

Skin rolling

The fingertips and thumbs are used. Grab about an inch (5 cm) of superficial fascia, pulling it away from the filmy and deeper fascia and making quick, rolling movements each time. This technique works well where the flesh is loose.

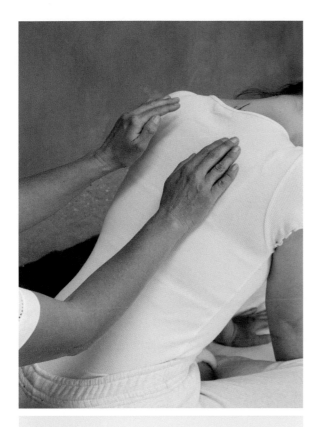

Fig. 20.4
Dtee Using hands this way provides a different sensation and a very hollow sound.

Rotations

These can be given with the heel of the hand, fingertips, or knuckles. This is a particularly effective technique for working the second layer of the body to release tension, softening and waking it up. If the heel of the hand is being used, place it on the body and then lean some weight on to that area. The hand should stay in the same place for a few rotations, moving the superficial fascia over the filmy fascia, before sliding to another position and repeating until

the whole region has been covered thoroughly. This technique lends itself well to certain areas such as the shoulders and gluteal muscles.

Compressions

These can be carried out with feet, hands, knees, elbows, shins, or any other area that is easy to lean on while maintaining balance. Each provides a different type of surface: some broader like the palm of a hand or sole of a foot (Fig. 20.5), others more focused, such as an elbow. Compressions are used as a way to work on the muscle and fascia. They are long, slow, deep holds that target one area at a time (Figs 20.6 and 20.7). Each compression is held

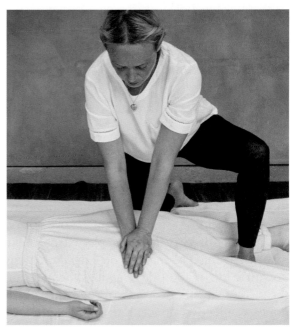

Fig. 20.5
The hand providing a long and slow compression to a tight, bound-up quadriceps.

Chapter 20

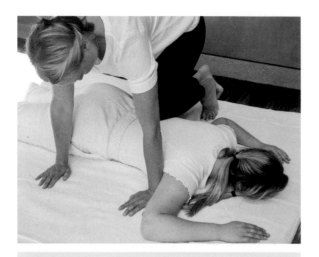

Fig. 20.6
Knees can provide really deep compressions without much effort from the practitioner.

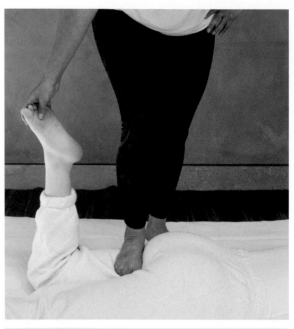

Fig. 20.7
The hamstrings can take deep pressure, as they are big muscles. The arch of the foot fits perfectly over the bulk of the muscle in this position and the practitioner can effortlessly use gravity to lean in. The recipient's toes are held to ensure the muscles are in a relaxed state before being compressed.

until the layer lets go of tension. It is patient work for the practitioner.

Transition to compressions

As well as being more pleasant to receive, easing in and out of deep compressions gives the practitioner time to feel the body. Being precise and focused on what is happening to the texture of that layer ensures that accurate pressure is applied. Sliding the hand, knee, forearm, or any other body part from one place to the next involves lifting it so that it is no longer applying pressure, but maintaining enough contact for the receiver to still be aware of your touch. It is not easy, effective, or accurate to slide and keep applying pressure at the same time.

Sometimes, especially for those people with Fire core element, long, slow, and deep compressions work best (Fig. 20.8). At other times – for example, when someone is fragile or in pain – it may be that a gentle com-

pression, held for shorter timeframes, is used. Either way, sinking in and out again is necessary. Make sure you remember that the body is not going to respond well to a sudden touch.

Palm gliding

This can be carried out with palms spread wide. The tissue is simultaneously pressed and pushed, repeatedly gliding the hands along the whole length of an area. The technique is used for relaxing muscles that are sore and tense (see spinal nerve treatment in Chapter 22).

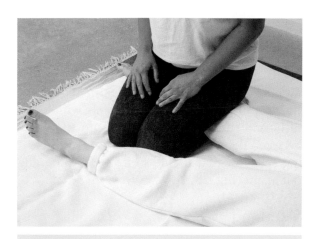

Fig. 20.8
The whole lower leg can be compressed in one go with this clever technique. The practitioner can adjust how much of their body weight they apply to ensure that the depth is adjusted to suit client needs.

Knuckle gliding

The hands are made into a fist and the knuckles used to glide on skin, giving a broad and strong touch (see spinal nerve treatment in Chapter 22).

Ironing

Thumbs or fingers are used. Balms and liniments lubricate the surface of the skin to allow for gliding, pressing, and pushing, but this variation gives a less broad, more direct touch, working repeatedly into the channels. This technique works on softening the tissue and Sên, and helps move Wind (see spinal nerve treatment in Chapter 22).

Stripping

This is the same technique as ironing but with a stretch or torsion applied to the tissue layer and Sên concurrently. It can consist of small and precise movements – for example, between the metacarpals of the hand – or a limb can be stretched and then worked on.

Wringing

There are many different versions of this technique, depending on the area that is being worked. It involves holding the tissue with two hands that work in opposite directions to each other, as if wringing out a rag. This frees up stuck tissue and, if it is performed on a hand or foot, can realign the bony structures.

Ban

Ban is a Thai word for a technique that involves agitating and vibrating an area. It mainly applies

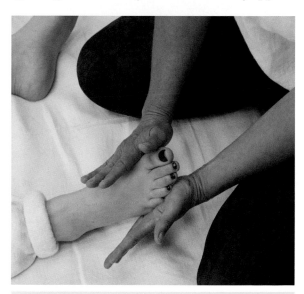

Fig. 20.9
Ban translates literally as "shake." It is used to help the foot joints realign, and as a vibrational technique to disperse stagnation.

to working on a foot, ankle, wrist, or hand. It can help small structures (like the 26 bones of the foot, the 131 joints in the foot or the 27 bones of a hand) move and then reorganize themselves. To take the foot as an example, the outside edges of the first and fifth metatarsal bones are held between the practitioner's palms. The hands stay in one place, not sliding on the skin but moving, forwards and back, and alternating with a steady but fast speed. This can also be carried out at the rear and mid foot (Fig. 20.9).

Dragging

This is performed by fingers, which are used to drag and pull tissue away from bone in one area repeatedly. Dragging makes space around a joint, freeing up stuck tissue and moving Wind element (Fig. 20.10).

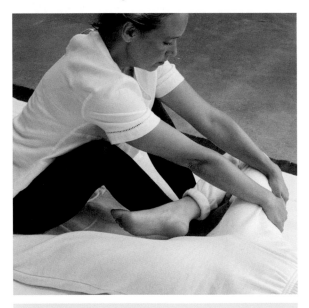

Fig. 20.10
The feet act as stabilizers and provide counterpressure, enabling the practitioner's hands to drag tissue strongly away from bone.

Digging

This is a way of getting right into tissue in one direction, using fingers or thumbs before digging the tissue back out again. If we take the scapula as an example, it feels wonderful to have a thumb pressed right into the space between the spine and scapula. Yet this is closing space in that tissue, so it needs to be dug out again (Fig. 20.11).

Scooping

Scooping is similar to digging but the focus is more on the channels. The thumbs or fingers create space using direction to push out or pull back.

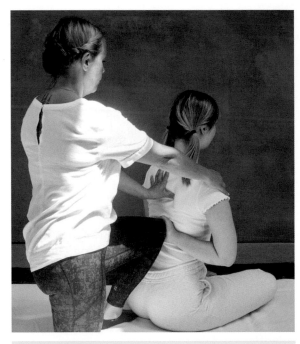

Fig. 20.11
Digging is a medial move to create space away from bone.

Fumbling

This technique is applied to areas around joints, specifically knees, elbows, wrists, and ankles. It creates space in the tissue layer, with the soft tissue sliding over the filmy fascia around these areas. The practitioner uses flat fingers to grasp just above or around the joint and makes circular motions (Fig. 20.12).

Stretching

Stretching is good for people who are stiff and tense, and for whom range of motion is limited or below what is healthy or natural for them. A huge variety of stretches can be performed and they mostly target a specific group of muscles (Figs 20.13 and 20.14; see Chapter 14 for more details).

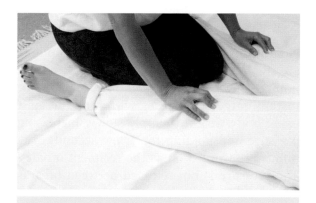

Fig. 20.12
Fingers are used to create space around the knee joints by working with the sliding surface of the perifascia.

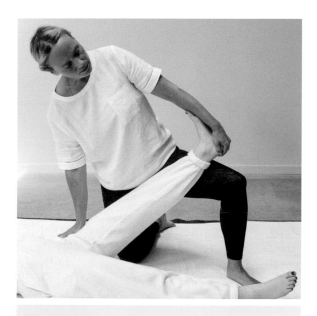

Fig. 20.13
A simple stretch of the calf muscle and plantar fascia.

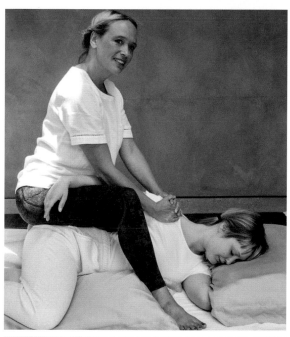

Fig. 20.14
Stretching the shoulders and neck in side-lying.

Chapter 20

Release points

Neuro-muscular and myofascial trigger points are the Western terms for these same release points. They can be worked on repeatedly for instant targeted release, with the therapist using body weight to apply slowly increasing pressure and holding for a few seconds. The points are worked on as the recipient inhales. The pressure is not released between breaths but is held as the recipient breathes out. This is repeated, pressing in further each time there is an inhalation. The points worked in Thai massage are located directly where the problem is; they do not distally refer (that is, if there is pain in the lumbar area of the back, this is where the points are) (Fig. 20.15).

Side note: Release points are located all over the body, commonly in the areas that we might refer to as "knots." They are, in fact, areas where the fascia has tightened or become bound up into a hardened form. They generally are caused by lack of nutritious movement, or poor and repeated function. Knuckles are used to apply pressure when working down between vertebrae or as a more general, broad touch.

Twisting

This is a way of getting passive movement and fluidity into the spine and other areas of the

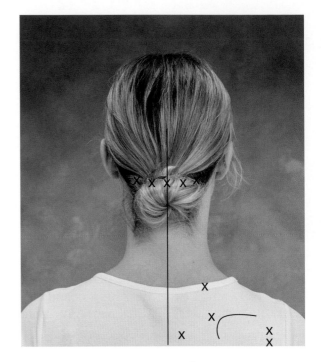

|_ Spine
| Scapula

X— Release points

Fig. 20.15
Location of shoulder and neck release points. They are similar to Western trigger points but do not distally refer.

body. There are a multitude of twists that the practitioner can choose from, and they target specific areas of the spine, side of the body, chest, and hips (Fig. 20.16).

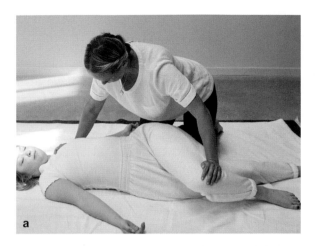

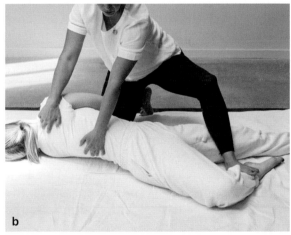

Fig. 20.16
Twisting. a. This targets the chest, front of body and lumbar spine. b. This targets the adductor muscles of the leg and the thoracic/lumbar spine.

Belly ball

This is an unusual technique, as it works the front and back of the body simultaneously. The practitioner uses flat hands on the abdomen and lower back to massage both areas. Belly ball also includes a gentle twist and the support of the practitioner's body.

Unwinding

Unwinding primarily concentrates on releasing the tissue layer of a limb. The tissue is grasped from one side and then pulled to the other. It might then be grasped from the opposite side and pulled back in the other direction. Each time, the tissue is being encouraged away from bone, making space. Generally, the fingers are used for this technique, although the forearm can be involved if working on a bigger muscle group like the quadriceps.

Scalp scrunches

These are performed only on the head. The practitioner grasps the hair in a clump at the root and skillfully clenches their fist. This creates a bit of space as it lifts up the scalp a little as the hair is pulled.

Pin and stretch

The practitioner will often stabilize or prevent one area from moving and take another into a stretch to accentuate and improve the efficacy of that particular move (Fig. 20.17).

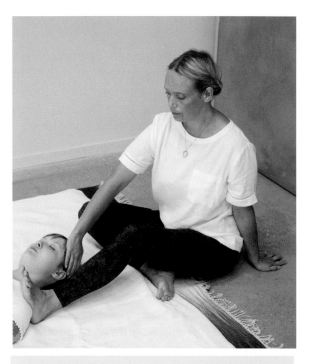

Fig. 20.17
The head is stabilized and the foot creates a stretch. A patient application of touch allows all the tiny muscle fibers to relax.

Khuut

Khuut is performed gently and repetitively with the edge of a tool (which must not be sharp). The purpose of this technique is to remove stagnation in the fascia and soft tissue, as well as to draw heat pathogens and toxins from deeper in the body to the skin so that the eliminatory function of the skin can process the work. The technique is found in many traditional practices around the world and has also been adopted in more recent years by Western manual therapy modalities with a focus on fascial release. The tool is used in a scooping motion.

When I first learned this technique, I used the edge of a lid, but since then I have also used a porcelain spoon and a special tool from a Chinese medicine shop that is made from bone (see Fig. 20.1). Chinese medicine uses the same technique and calls it Gua Sha. Traditionally, a horn would have been used.

Khuut is very effective for releasing tense and blocked areas where other techniques are not working, and is a powerful way to release heat toxins from the body and to manage pain. It tends to leave marks on the skin for a few days afterwards, but these are helpful for diagnosis of what is happening deeper in the body. It is surprisingly relaxing to receive, and clients often go into a deeply relaxed state, or sleep. It is good to let the client rest a while before standing up after Khuut has been performed and to encourage them to continue to rest and keep warm for a few hours after the session, as this technique releases a lot of heat. Due to it bringing up pathogens from deep within, the body needs time to deal with and process the response.

Tissue plucking

This technique can be used on the tissue layer or directly on gross Sên (Fig. 20.18). It involves grasping the tissue and quickly making an upward, snapping movement, before releasing. This is done with such speed that the upward movement and release happen almost simultaneously. It is repeated many times over until the tissue softens or tension

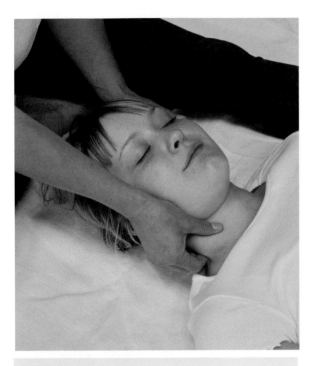

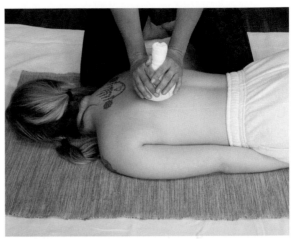

Fig. 20.19
Herbal compresses are an excellent tool for massage and a good way of getting medicinal herbs into the body via the skin.

Fig. 20.18
The anterior surface of the neck is a busy area for Sên. Tissue plucking can be used to address tension and as focused work for the brachial plexus.

around the Sên has slackened off. The depth of pressure varies according to the area being worked. For example, it will be very different around the sternocleidomastoid from around the Achilles tendon.

Cupping

This technique is not exclusive to Thai bodywork but can be seen in many cultures with traditional medicine. Cupping is traditionally performed with glass, ceramic, or metal cups, but nowadays can also be carried out with silicone for ease. This technique draws heat toxins and other pathogens from the deeper layers. It also creates space, and moves blood and Wind.

Herbal compresses

Due to the herbal ingredients, these tools are a great way to treat the layers. They can be strong and effective without deep application. The heat is soothing, relaxing, and opening. Compresses are hugely therapeutic and effective, as they can address all five layers of the body, depending on which herbs are in them (Fig. 20.19; see Chapter 15 for more detailed information).

Scarves

Scarves can be used to massage the body, and to provide traction and create space. They shake things up and get deep work done, combining the depth of the work with movement. They are useful in many specific areas of the body, such as the lumbar spine and neck.

Fascial stretching

This can release a joint and the shorter muscles that surround that joint. It is particularly beneficial if there is stiffness, immobility, or areas that have gone into spasm. It can also target the perifascial layer, the practitioner moving tissue in opposite directions and focusing on the sliding surface beneath the superficial fascia. This type of stretching concentrates on fascial connections and can be applied to smaller areas, targeting them specifically to release pain (Fig. 20.20).

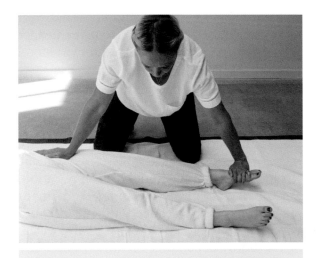

Fig. 20.20
Fascial stretching focuses primarily on the second layer.

Muscle resistance technique

This is commonly known in the West as "muscle energy technique" (MET). Simply put, a stretch is applied to an area against the exertion of the recipient, which activates neuro-muscular activity. The practitioner actively holds the stretch and asks the recipient to push against them while breathing in. As the pressure is released, the recipient relaxes the breath and the effort (Fig. 20.21).

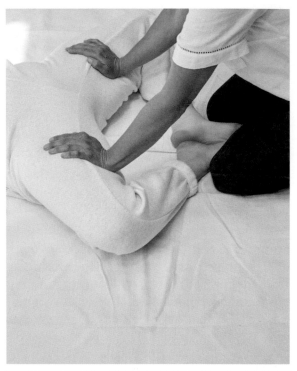

Fig. 20.21
The recipient pushes up against the downward pressure of the practitioner's hands before the technique is released and reapplied.

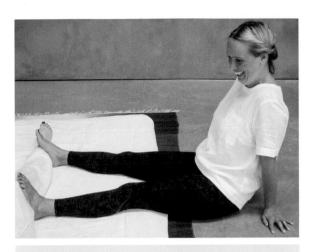

Fig. 20.22
Using the outside edge of the foot to intensify depth of pressure without the therapist straining or working hard.

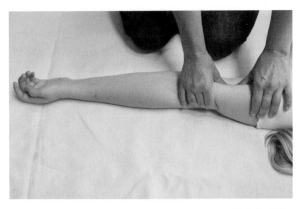

Fig. 20.23
Clearing the channels on the arm to stimulate the Sên.

Blading

The outside edge of the foot is used to increase the level of pressure that is being applied as the hardness of bone is utilized (Fig. 20.22). It is the foot appendage equivalent of forearm rolling.

Channels

Thumb pressing

This is well known and much used throughout Thai bodywork. Sometimes, if the area needs intricate touch, fingertips are used. Otherwise, it is the flat of the thumb that applies pressure to the grooves (located between muscles, or between muscle and bone), with the practitioner working to encourage space and stimulate the underlying Sên.

Thumb pressing involves placing one thumb on top of the other, or working with the thumbs side by side (tips touching). Thumbs are the primary tool for working the channels and Sên, although elbows and fingers can be used too. Which you choose depends on the size, space, and location of the channels, and the size of the practitioner in relation to the patient.

The practitioner leans weight on to the thumbs, sinking slowly in, then slowly releases and slides the thumbs by moving them two knuckles, length further up or down the channel being worked (Fig. 20.23).

There are three variations for working the channels. The first is to work directionally and involves always working in that same direction to move Wind. The other two are carried out with thumbs being pressed up and down the channels in both directions. The second way involves greater focus on stimulating the Sên, moving up and down a channel to input touch repeatedly to the pathways of movement deep to the fascia. The third creates more space in the fascia, which frees up the underlying Sên (see Chapter 10).

Elbow pressing

This is used for deep pressure into the channels and is helpful when precise sustained pressure is needed. It can be valuable for release point work (Fig. 20.24).

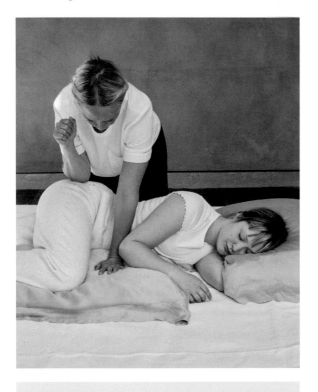

Fig. 20.24
Using the olecranon process to work into the channels around the sacrum and posterior superior iliac spine.

Thumb ironing

This alternative to thumb pressing is mainly used with an application of oil. Thumbs are placed on top of each other and glide along the trenches repetitively to work into and soften them. It moves Wind element and releases tension.

Elbow ironing

This is a variation where the elbow is used instead of the thumb to glide repetitively along the channels. It is used for directional work – for example, where there is an injury – and application of a medicinal balm moves Wind away from the site of pain.

Sên

Wind Gate

Working the Wind Gates (see Chapter 22) is a wonderful technique if performed with skill. It can be carried out in areas such as the top of the femur, the abdomen, and the armpits. Wind Gate work involves slowly and gently engaging with the pulses. Performing this technique with a lot of care and attention is a powerful way to release and encourage movement of Wind in areas where it is stuck, much like opening a gate (hence the name).

Sfln plucking

This targets gross Sên, such as the sciatic nerve, sternocleidomastoid, and Achilles tendon. Depth of pressure, grasp, and speed will depend on the individual and the structure being worked on. For example, plucking the Achilles would be much stronger work than plucking the sternocleidomastoid, which would be worked on with a focus on releasing the vagus nerve from its surrounding tissue.

Joints

Stagnation around the joints is common, as they are problem areas in the body, places where things become stuck and create pain. It is important to address them properly in a session. Often, the muscle and soft tissue around the joint need softening and working on before reaching this (bone) layer. Thai massage and bodywork can go a long way towards helping people with pain in their joints. A broad approach will encompass the use of medicinal balms and liniments, herbal compresses, passive movement, and stretching to work the whole area. There are three primary techniques that get these areas moving: range of motion, vibration, and traction.

Imagine the joints as busy, congested areas; when they hurt, they are a bit like traffic on a busy road that has come to a standstill. Nothing can move, traffic is piling up, and the knock-on effects of this congestion are far-reaching. The same applies to the body. If there is a problem in one joint, the whole of the rest of the body somehow compensates, doing a brilliant job of functioning as best it can. Time after time, I see familiar patterns: the neck and lower back have an intimate relationship, as do the shoulders and hips (which function as a unit – take note of how we swing the opposite arm to leg when walking to maintain balance). The positioning of the ankle can affect the temporomandibular joint, and so on.

Range of motion

This is used for the bone layer, so ideally should be worked on after the skin, muscle, and Sên layers. There are times when the Sên have not been worked but the joints still benefit from being taken through their natural ranges to passively bring movement to that area (Fig. 20.25). If you are doing this, it is much more beneficial if the first and second layers have already been worked to warm up the tissues around the joint.

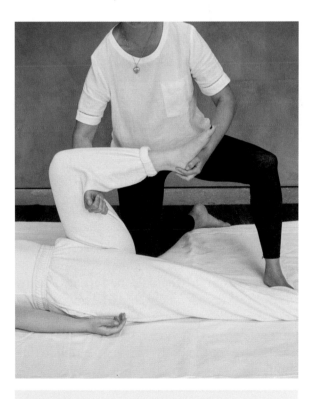

Fig. 20.25
Range of motion encourages synovial fluid and stagnation to move.

Adjustments to the joints often inadvertently happen as a natural response to soft tissue release, a natural self-realignment without any force.

Each joint can be taken through any or all of its natural ranges (on the sagittal, transverse, or frontal plane) to encourage better movement, and to release toxins that can easily be stored in these areas. It is important to know which movements a joint makes, rather than try to force it into an unnatural range.

The range of motion techniques are carried out to get things moving again. There is often a build-up of stagnated synovial fluids in the bends of the body. The range of motion techniques help to clear these stuck areas. They move accumulated Wind and lubricate the joint through movement (all movement is hydrating). The repetitions should be carried out many times, paying attention to the body and what it needs. The nearby joints should also be worked in a directional way to move the Wind.

Traction

This is a technique for the bone layer. For it to be effective and create a change in the soft tissue around the joint, it should be repeated many times (traditionally, between nine and twenty-one). Traction involves slowly pulling a limb or joint away from the body. As this addresses the fourth layer of the body, this is a technique that should be carried out after the three preceding layers have been addressed (Fig. 20.26).

Vibration

Vibration shakes things up to banish stagnation (Fig. 20.27).

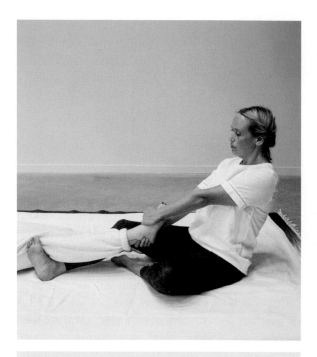

Fig. 20.26
Traction can be performed with scarves or hands. It is a technique that creates space between two areas where stagnation has built up.

Balms and Liniments

Balms are made with oil, liniments with alcohol. Both are applied to the skin with the focus on getting the herbs into the body to provide healing. Unlike Western massage modalities, the balm or liniment is applied and worked into the skin layer, then reapplied again and again until the herbs have really been absorbed and can effect a change. Depending on the recipe, the product could penetrate any or all layers.

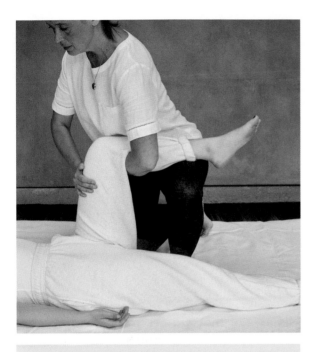

Fig. 20.27
Vibration gets stagnation moving and is carried out on all the joints in the body individually. The application changes, depending on which joint is being targeted.

Esoteric Practices

Jit Jai

Jit Jai is the practice of gently thumb-pressing and stimulating specific points located throughout the body, and calms or nourishes the heart–mind. It can calm the mental Winds, anxiety, disturbing thoughts, a broken heart, palpitations, brain fog, and any problem that involves the heart and mind being agitated.

The heart and mind are seen as one thing, as you can see in the translation of each word:

- Jit is "mind/heart/thoughts."

- Jai is "heart/mind/spirit" (Thai2english. com).

There is a pulse in the thumb called the princeps pollicis artery and it is Sên. This big artery is the reason that traditional Thai practitioners (and allopathic doctors in the West) do not use the thumb to feel a pulse, as it will be misleading for diagnosis; it is, however, used for Jit Jai work because it sends Winds to the points (Fig. 20.28).

Spirit Medicine

Tok Sfln

This involves the practitioner using a mallet and peg to gently and repetitively tap along channels, sending a vibration to the Sên. While this is a technique for the central nervous system, it is also spirit medicine, as the practitioner silently repeats a healing incantation throughout the treatment. This tool is often used to drive away spirits that are causing suffering.

Tool cleansing

Sompoy water, with or without turmeric (dry or fresh), can be used to clean Tok Sên, scraping and cupping tools, and as the water for Chet and Haek (spirit medicine). This cleansing water also serves as a wash for the practitioner's body after treatments.

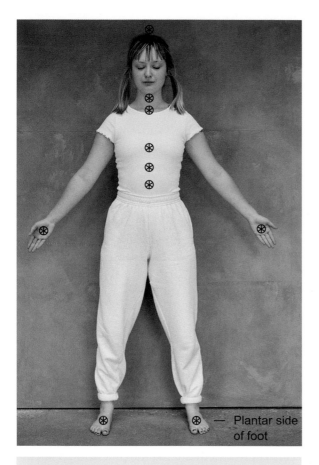

Fig. 20.28
Jit Jai. The heart and mind are seen as one in Thai medicine. The depth of pressure that stimulates these points is subtle.

Plantar side of foot

Sompoy cleans negative energies, and protects against spirits and ghosts. It also increases the power of incantations and imbues the tools with extra healing powers.

The water should have the herbs added to it and be left to sit for at least half an hour before being used. It should be changed at the end of each day.

Side note: Sompoy's Latin name is *Acacia concinna*, and in English it is called soap nut.

Uses of spirit medicine

Diseases of the skin are traditionally treated with cupping, smokes and steams, and herbal formulas applied topically.

The Sên are treated with herbal formulas (ingested in the form of infusions, decoctions, and medicine), therapeutic bodywork, and compresses with herbs that penetrate the first three layers of the body.

Blood is treated through internal herbal formulas, blood-letting and wet-cupping. This last is a technique whereby toxic blood is drawn to the surface with cups, the skin is lightly cut, and the toxic blood is released from the body. It is found in many traditional cultures and is a specialized treatment requiring professional training and instruction.

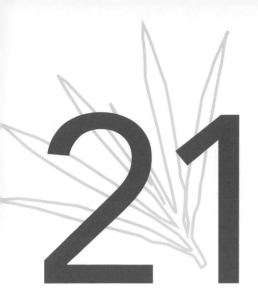

21 Putting It All Together

The general goal of Thai massage is to create enough space in the soft tissues that the Winds can move freely through the body.

At the beginning, I recommend starting out with a basic sequence that cares thoroughly for each textural layer and ensures that the recipient's body is treated with integrity, sinking or melting slowly through the layers in a patient way with awareness.

For each area:

- *Skin* – rubbing/warming.

- *Palpation* (some practitioners prefer to palpate before rubbing and then again after rubbing) – feeling, sensing, and ascertaining which area(s) need(s) to be worked on.

- *Soft tissue layer* – choosing two or three techniques for each area and using them repeatedly (compression, forearm roll, squeeze, dragging, stretching).

- *Channel and Sên layer* – if the body feels ready, indicated by the malleability of the soft tissue in that area.

- *Bone layer* – range of motion, vibration, and traction (nine or more times each as

a minimum, ideally until the joint feels lubricated and free).

It is important to establish the priority for the treatment on any particular day so that the client gets the most out of the session. You can also determine a secondary issue, so that if you have time, you can move on to that. Working this way, rather than trying to cover the whole body, will actually relax and benefit the recipient much more because it releases the area that most needs it. This is extremely therapeutic and what most people's bodies are crying out for, especially when pain is getting them down.

As a general rule of thumb, you can work on:

- one area during a 1-hour session

- two areas in 1.5 hours

- two areas and some more general work in 2 hours.

Thai medical theory is highly complex. There are so many factors to take into account that it can become overwhelming, and I often see students and practitioners becoming confused about how to put it all into practice. For this reason, I am going to provide an overview of treatments I have carried out as a loose guide

Chapter 21

to get you going; they are examples, case studies only. However, there are so many variables that they must be taken as a springboard, and not by any means considered definitive. Some of what I do in treatments may involve using tools that you have not yet been initiated in or given instructions for, and may be out of your current skill set. Most important is that the practitioner broadens and widens their own knowledge and sees as many people as possible to develop confidence and efficacy with their current skill set and the techniques they have been taught.

Ancient Knowledge

One of my teachers, a Reusi, is a guardian of the knowledge of Thai medicine, and has amassed information from a long line of teachers, village doctors, Reusi, and monks. The importance he places on maintaining the traditions comes from a deep reverence for his teachers and for Buddhism. He stresses the importance of learning Buddha Dhamma, as this is where the elements, the layers of the body, the eightfold path, the four noble truths, and many more teachings of the Buddha bring to light some of the theory that underlies this modality as Buddhist medicine.

Successful Bodywork

Being a successful therapeutic bodywork practitioner comes from investing in studying, and I believe that to have a good basis this study should include theory, the body, the elements, movement, connectivity, links between the heart, gut, and mind, the web of fascial continuity, and dissection. To achieve good results in clinic and to run a practice that is fulfilling and successful, there must also be reflection, observation, willingness to go deep into study, and continuous curiosity.

If practitioners of Thai bodywork started treating using set sequences and handling everyone in the same way, a large part of the efficacy of the work would be lost and the traditional approach would not be honored. Therapeutic work needs a practitioner who takes the pulse, provides a comprehensive consultation, thinks through the variables, and tailors the session each time. Whatever treatment is performed, it is essential for the layers of the body to be cared for; this is absolute basic-level practice and will ensure the safe practice and effectiveness of your work. The body is sacred and should be treated as such. Have awareness that, when applying bodywork, you need to be invited and welcomed in, rather than forcing your way like an intruder. Thai massage can be deep, and with respect for the textural layers, patient work, and the correct choice of tools for the presenting symptoms, it has huge healing potential.

Side note: A practitioner should spend time reflecting on their practice, and have patience and dedication to learning what each individual body needs, rather than learning how to treat. Essentially, this means studying theory, rather than just learning more techniques. Much of this comes with time.

A treatment might be performed in a clinic environment, when a set time has been planned and booked, but equally it could be that you are giving a family member, neighbor, or friend a session on the kitchen floor to alleviate their pain, when you both have ten minutes to spare and kids and animals are coming in and out of the space. The work lends itself to any environment and this is why (along with the use of everyday herbs for internal and external healing work) it could be seen as "kitchen medicine" (Fig. 21.1).

In practice, a session is never repeated: each and every session will vary and be tailored to what is best suited to help someone heal. I have tried to give an outline of the conditions I see frequently in my clinic, and a summary of what might go through my mind as I decide how to proceed with the session. This is by no means exhaustive, as there are many variables when working with people.

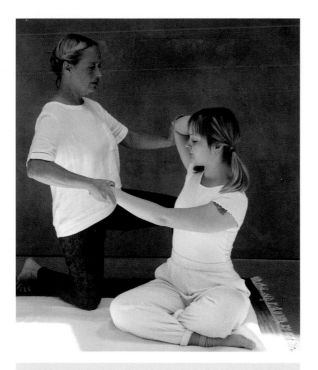

Fig. 21.1
One of the most common traditional positions for the delivery of Thai massage is seated on the floor.

Another point I would like to make is related to being cautious, and to the questions that come from this approach. It is better to err on the side of caution and be able to look back and say that you could have done more, rather than take a treatment too far and cause harm. I would say that this is especially true when seeing a client for the first few treatments as you get to know each other.

Side note: For a practitioner, reflection is key: thinking through the treatment process, the choices you made, the techniques you performed, the conversations you had, the pressure you applied, and so on.

Choices

When formulating a treatment plan, it is really important for the practitioner to make choices that are tailored to the current needs of the client. Absolutely every technique, tool, direction, and component of the treatment should be employed because it is what they need at that particular moment. This is because it is the best way to achieve the desired treatment outcomes (and ensure that satisfied clients return). It is much more effective to repeat techniques until a change has occurred than to constantly change from one to another. It is work requiring patience. For this reason, it is important to really know what you are doing and why.

Adjusting to the Client's Needs

It is very common for a practitioner to give a treatment that they would like to receive personally, and this can be problematic. I have observed this many times with students, and when I point it out they are immediately able to notice what they are doing. For example, a typically CEC Windy practitioner who has a preference for being treated with care (slow, measured, melting work) will probably irritate the CEC Fiery type who wants the pressure to go deep quickly and with a definite, confident, "get in there" approach.

A Fiery practitioner most definitely needs to tone things down if the roles are reversed and they are working on a sensitive and Windy person, especially if their Winds are agitated. The fast pace and intense pressure will really aggravate or even upset a Windy person, making them more anxious and chaotic, and this will be counterproductive. This aspect of the treatment is important to have in your mind as you work because it is another layer of attention to detail that will make all the difference to the treatment outcome and will produce a returning, happy, and satisfied client who will go on to refer others to you.

Pulse Diagnosis

Five-limb pulse diagnosis is a really useful diagnostic tool that, if your training allows, will help ascertain where the Winds are blocked. It can also be used to diagnose the general state of elemental imbalance (Water, Fire, and Wind) (Fig. 21.2; see Chapter 20).

Working Directionally

The practitioner can work to encourage the Wind's direction and to set things moving therapeutically. If someone is very anxious and "up in their head," it is best to work directionally away from the head towards the feet and the stable element of the Earth. If a client

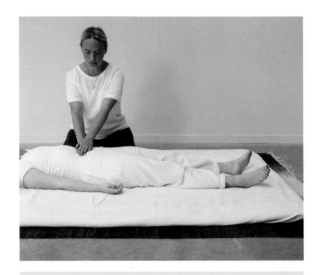

Fig. 21.2
The navel Wind Gate is also the mother pulse and is a diagnostic tool.

is weak and fatigued, and low in Fire, it is helpful to work towards the core, to bring as much vitality there as possible. If there is an injury, work away from it to disperse it in all directions. If the problem is that someone is overflowing with energy and cannot calm down, it is best to work from the core to the limbs, dispersing their Fire to the rest of the body.

Why Working on One Area Will Help Another

In Thai medical theory, Sên do not distally refer, unlike the meridians in Chinese medicine. This is because Sên are physical components of the body. If an area hurts, the release points will be located directly at or around the area of pain. However, there is often a sensation and release in distal areas, explained by the Winds moving through pathways from one place to another. The continuity and connectivity from superficial to deep, and from one end of the body to another, are other factors: no one area is separate from another.

Spinal nerves leave the spinal column between the vertebrae, with each individual nerve root traveling to its own specific area of the skin, which it innervates, giving sensory feedback. The area of the skin that each nerve corresponds to is called a **dermatome**. A **myotome** is a group of muscles that is controlled and acted on by a single spinal nerve. If we think about these from the viewpoint of Thai medicine, it would consider the communication as being along Sên, pathways of movement from deep to superficial. It is important to note that this example is used to highlight the Winds moving through the body, rather than being a description that would be found in Thai medical texts, with the aim of helping us understand why we experience relief in places far away from the input of touch.

Working with Oils, Balms, and Liniments

It goes without saying that a Thai bodyworker will at some point (usually fairly early on in training) want to include some of the herbal roots of Thai medicine in their work. There is a variety of specific medicinal oils, balms, and liniments that promote healing and that address, support, or nourish conditions and imbalances (Fig. 21.3).

The Thai physical therapist uses herbs in many forms so that their medicinal properties can work on the body. Floral waters (such as rose or jasmine) are soothing and calming to the mental Winds. There are many recipes in the books listed in the Resources section later. In these, colleagues have documented ancient

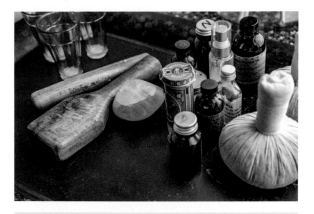

Fig. 21.3
Medicinal herbal balms, liniments, and compresses are an essential part of a toolkit. The wooden mallet and peg are a bodywork and spirit medicine tool called Tok Sên. With kind permission of Katie Bracher.

and also more recent recipes, some handed down originally from village doctors in Northern Thailand, some coming from their own personal tutors, and some being found in ancient Thai traditional medical books. These recipes are often labor-intensive and take real patience to make, but they are truly amazing when used in the right circumstances, giving extra health-promoting efficacy to the bodywork.

A huge selection of balms, liniments, creams, and oils can be applied directly to the skin and massaged in. The practitioner works the product into the body using rubbing, kneading, gliding, ironing, and other such techniques, and as it absorbs into the body it will be reapplied repeatedly, with the purpose of helping the herbs penetrate thoroughly. Using these products, the Thai practitioner takes a different approach to Western styles because the application is repeated many times. For example, when implementing the spinal nerve protocol, a nerve liniment is used. This particular recipe addresses the physical nerves while also being calming and soothing.

Side note: Coconut oil can be used to subdue Fire element, as it is slightly more cooling than other oils. Raw sesame oil is warming. Castor oil is drawing.

Case Studies

In these case studies I have listed the main concerns that needed treatment, rather than giving the whole client history. I list symptoms rather than giving labels, as this encourages us to move away from Western diagnosis and toward a tailored Thai therapeutic treatment session.

Side note: Please remember that these are not prescriptions for treatments, but are a snapshot of possible ways to work. There are so many variations that arise through the consultation process, observation, and experience.

As I have already explained, I will usually try to address one area of concern in 1 hour, two areas of concern in 1.5 hours, and two areas of concern plus some more general treatment in 2 hours. I rarely try to address the whole body, as the session is unlikely to be thorough if it attempts to cover such a large area therapeutically. A whole-body massage is usually performed for relaxation purposes alone. The practitioner would decide on this being the therapeutic treatment if it were going to be of most benefit over and above any other work.

Conversely, the focus on painful and symptomatic areas is wonderfully relaxing, and most people who are suffering want the treatment to concentrate on the area of concern rather than being a more general massage.

The areas focused on are highlighted in *italic* type.

Case Study 1 (2 hours)

Anxious pretty much all the time. *Lower back* is aching, especially on the left side. Head feels muzzy and *foggy*. *Neck* is sore at occipital ridge, caused by too much time at the computer. Completely *exhausted*. Main concerns are neck, back, and energy levels.

Supine

Start at the head and work directionally towards the core to nourish her.

Massage the scalp and face intensively with a focus on relaxation to address the anxiety. Jasmine floral water to help calm the mental Winds and release point work around the crown to ease the fogginess.

Neck massage with hot herbal compresses and then plai cream, which is especially good for the skin, muscle, and soft tissue layers.

Strong work around the occiput and sagittal work from the forehead to occiput, concentrating on opening and creating space for fluids to drain here (this is a natural drainage system in the body and also a channel).

Herbal compresses around the sternum and pectoral muscles, followed by heel into pectoral muscles with slow, patient, and melting application.

The pectoral muscles have a direct link to the sternocleidomastoid muscles of the anterior neck and so need physical therapy to help release the tension in the neck.

Pin and stretch, using the foot and holding the head.

Cervical spine channels to address the Sên.

Scarf work to massage the neck deeply and provide traction to the fourth layer.

Prone

Hot herbal compresses, used slightly wet to address and calm her agitated Wind imbalance, which was showing as pain and anxiety.

Back – second layer – forearm rolls, deep compressions, deep compressions with heel on shoulders (Fig. 21.4). Crossed-hand fascial stretching on back and on spine. Muscle and sacro-iliac joint traction of the lower back (Fig. 21.5).

Spinal nerve treatment with nerve oil (to calm the mental Winds and physical nerves). This treatment also helps when someone is below par and, with a downward (inferior) repetitive direction of techniques, encourages the flow of blood, cerebrospinal fluid, and energy away from head, where it is already busy.

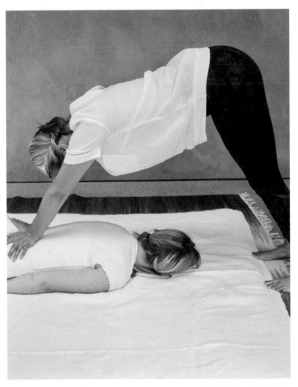

Fig. 21.5
An effective stretch technique which creates space between the lumbar spine and sacro-iliac joint using the practitioner's body weight.

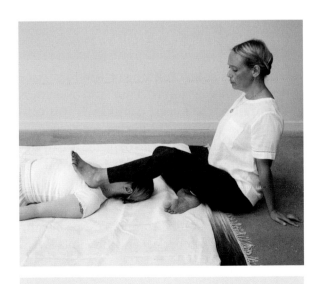

Fig. 21.4
The heel has to melt slowly into the soft tissue and can be used for effective and deep work.

Supine

Nerve oil on feet and hands with massage and traction of the fingers and toes. The slow-pulling traction calms the nervous system and nerve oil can be used to balance Wind.

Case Study 2 (2 hours)

Had been suffering from lower *back weakness* caused by over-exercise, then sneezed in bed and back went into *spasm*. Since then, has not been able to stand or sit, as feels there is no strength in back to hold him up. *Numbness* in right *quad, hip, calf,* and *foot.* Finding it hard to move his toes without a lot of concentration. *Sexual dysfunction.*

This was a good example of using Thai element theory to make treatment choices and an opportunity to put to one side the more obvious Western diagnosis of "sciatica." My understanding of "sciatica" is that it affects each person differently, so it is always important to establish the individual somatic experience, considering the symptoms and not the diagnosis. This client was in considerable acute pain and fearful of movement. I wanted to stimulate and awaken the Sên but was aware the muscle layer was in spasm due to on-going pain.

Side-lying

This was the most restful position, using pillows to support his body and help him be comfortable.

I worked for a long time with hot herbal compresses on his back and legs to warm and relax the tissue layer, letting the herbs penetrate deeper to the Sên, using a specific recipe for Sên/nerves.

Prone

Rubbing first, using a heating oil at a stimulating pace to wake up the nerves. Following this, I used nerve oil repeatedly down the channels that lie next to the spine, known as the laminar groove.

Tok Sên on his back to work on the Sên with vibration, which is gentle but penetrates through the layers and directly influences nerves.

I worked on the right leg with techniques such as kneading, squeezing, and beating, to disperse the tension of the muscle layer, as well as more compresses.

I used heating liniments again in the channels of his legs. My goal was to do as much work as I could on the Sên, plucking and digging around the sciatic nerve and into the channels as much as possible, working down towards and including the right foot.

Case Study 3 (1.5 hours)

Knee pain caused by running on a hard surface with *hypermobile* joints. Pain and weakness at the front of the knees. Considered this case elementally – agitated Wind element (too much movement in the joints) and depleted Earth element (causing instability). All pain is Wind.

Supine

Used slightly wet herbal compresses specifically for penetrating to muscle, Sên, and joints layer.

Bent the leg to use compresses on the posterior leg.

Worked on the knee itself with compresses and massaged injury liniment into the patella and structures all around the patella (anterior and posterior) directionally and repeatedly.

Worked up the leg from the knee to the hip joint, and down the leg from the knee to ankle and foot: that is, away from the injured area.

Feet on hamstring, seated calf compression, feet on ilio-tibial band with blading, deep compressions around quads.

Stabilizing joint stretches (Fig. 21.6).

Wind Gates at inguinal crease to settle Winds.

Range of motion, traction, and vibration of whole leg.

Case Study 4 (1.5 hours)

Insomnia, along with *anxiety* and high *stress* levels. Finding it hard to get to sleep and waking in the early hours, then unable to get back to sleep; mind is racing. Feels *low in energy* and lacking enthusiasm. On observation, this client had a noticeable wild look in her eyes, almost like panic, telling me her body was in a state of fight or flight.

Supine

Placed herbal compresses on abdomen, asking client to move them when necessary.

Massage of head and scalp. Covered eyes with hands and held for a few minutes.

Massaged ears and covered ears with hands to promote relaxation and calm the Winds.

Face and neck massage with herbal compresses, followed by floral rose water on the face, the soothing scent being used to calm the central nervous system.

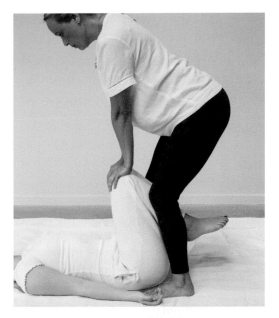
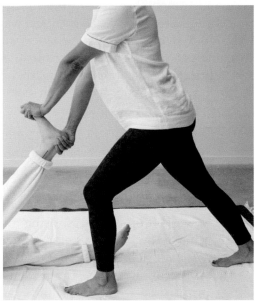

Fig. 21.6
a. Stabilizing the sacrum and knee joints.
b. Stabilizing the ankle, knee, and hip joints.

Nerve oil in the paravertebral trough on the cervical spine in an inferior direction.

Eight-finger hold at the occiput with slight traction and pressure on release points.

Wind Gates to settle nervous system.

Heart–mind points.

Prone

Herbal compress on back.

Spinal nerve treatment to calm the nerves.

Case Study 5 (1.5 hours)

Tired legs that have puffed up and become watery and dimply. Leg *sore* to the touch all over. Aching *lower back*. Legs never feel warm but the cold is also making them feel sore. Heavy, lifeless. *Skin* is *very sensitive* to any touch, fabric feels uncomfortable against her skin. Feet have been in agony with *crystal-sharp pain* areas, anterior and posterior.

This treatment was to move the stagnated fluids towards the abdomen, where the organs could process the work. The puffiness, tenderness, and cold of her legs meant she was very sensitive to touch, and even gentle palpation was sore. I worked on both legs, using all of these techniques on one leg before moving to the other. I started with the leg that was less sore on palpation because the movement of fluids on this leg would help fluids move through her whole system, so that when I started on the second leg she would already be processing the therapeutic work. Choosing to work on the less sore leg also built trust and helped her nervous system settle.

Supine

Hot herbal compresses working directionally from feet to abdomen for a long time.

Used a faster speed to really set the fluids moving, but making sure the level of end-feel pressure was optimum for her and noting that, as her legs warmed up, she could tolerate deeper application of pressure with the compresses.

Rubbing skin.

Wringing out the feet (Fig. 21.7).

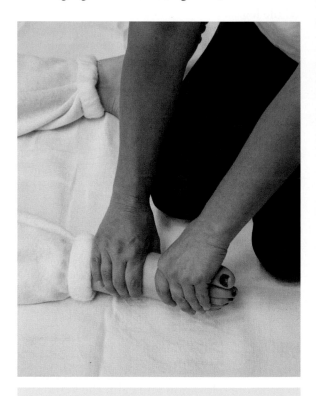

Fig. 21.7
Mobilizing the feet to help the thirty-three joints reorganize themselves.

Squeezing and kneading feet, then legs.

Ban on feet.

Dragging calf muscles with bent leg (Fig. 21.8).

Dragging and myofascial work on upper leg (Fig. 21.9).

Forearm rolling.

Beating.

Sitting on calves with pillows to compress tissue without too much pressure.

Femoral Wind Gate.

Range of motion, traction, and vibration.

Case Study 6 (1 hour)

Trigger thumb, tension in *shoulders* and *neck* from repeated long-distance driving (gripping the steering wheel), stress, and overwork (repetitive strain).

Trigger thumb was the priority with this treatment, so I worked directionally, moving the Winds in both directions throughout the treatment.

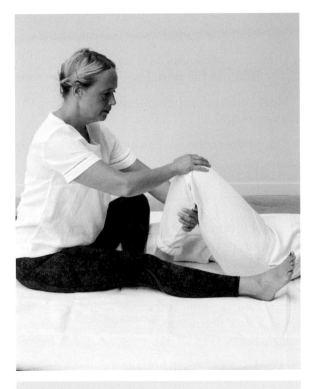

Fig. 21.8
Dragging tissue away from bone.

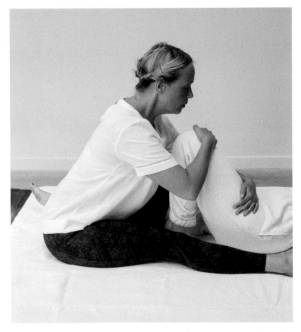

Fig. 21.9
The forearm and hand are used to drag the large muscles away from bone on the upper leg, which ensures correct body mechanics.

Supine

Herbal compresses from neck to hands in both directions.

Massage of the whole arm and hand with a warming balm (see Resources).

Khuut (scraping) of whole arm with directional work from shoulders to fingertips (Fig. 21.10).

Range of motion.

Drawing liniment (see Resources).

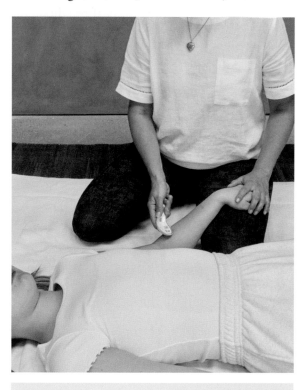

Fig. 21.10
A simple spoon is the perfect tool for this ancient Lanna technique called Khuut.

Case Study 7 (1 hour)

Restless legs that are worse at night but noticeable every time she sits down. Feels as if they are buzzing and makes her feel irritable all over. I wanted to get the Winds moving and calmed, and to address the Sên of the whole body by working on the spinal nerves.

Prone

Directional work from shoulders to feet with herbal compresses to warm and address layers.

Nerve oil and spinal nerve treatment.

Deep compressions held for long periods on legs – calming the muscles.

Nerve oil in channels on legs. Addressing the nerves directly.

Tok Sên on legs – to calm nerves with vibrational work.

Supine

Herbal compresses to address first and second layers, preparing the body for work on channels/Sên.

Feet on hamstrings to work second layer with deep compressions and create space where the muscle was bound up and pressing on to the sciatic nerve (Fig. 21.11).

Wind Gates, resetting the nervous system and calming the whole body.

Range of motion, traction, and vibration of leg and feet, to set the Winds moving.

Case Study 8 (2 hours)

Primary cause for concern was *headaches*, producing a gripping sensation at the forehead, with pain and tension radiating into *jaw* and *neck*. Described as constant, 24/7 for three days. Is a night jaw-clencher; condition is also stress- and work-related as has been sitting at a desk and driving a lot more than usual.

Supine

Close the eyes – this is very relaxing and puts gentle compression on the eye socket area.

Massage of the face and scalp for a long time using herbal compresses and hands. Herbal compresses placed around the neck, to be in position while working on the face and head.

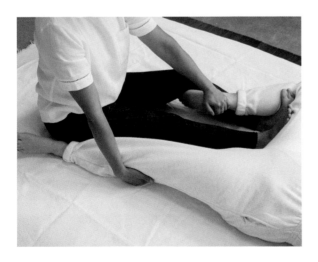

Fig. 21.11
Feet can be used in many ways to work deep into the large hamstring muscles and to do specific Sên release work.

Lots of first and second layer work and focus around the mandible, temporo-mandibular joint, digastric muscle, and jaw.

Used fingers and thumbs to work into all the spaces between bones around the face and head.

Scalp scrunches.

Release points on the face and head.

Massage of the ears, including pulling them in an inferior and lateral direction to create space – tissue away from bone.

Closing the ears – this creates a very relaxing inward focus and quiet, as it blocks out sound.

Massage of the suboccipitals.

Prone

Herbal compresses around shoulders and down back.

Heel on shoulders to ease tension there.

Slow compressions down the back to the sacrum.

Stretch to target the sacro-iliac joint, as the position of the pelvis is often related to the position of the frontal bone.

Seated

Two feet on the back to open chest as a counterpose to driving and computer work.

Massage of the posterior neck muscles using the arm (Fig. 21.12).

Case Study 9 (2 hours)

Hand tremors, sore neck, shoulders, and *back*, with *repetitive strain* on left elbow. Highly

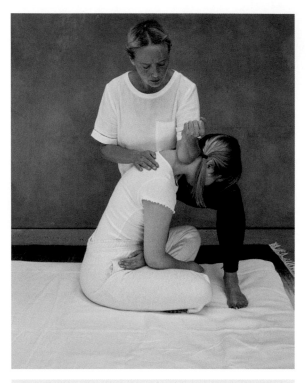

Fig. 21.12
The humerus is used to apply pressure and the practitioner's body is used as counterpressure.

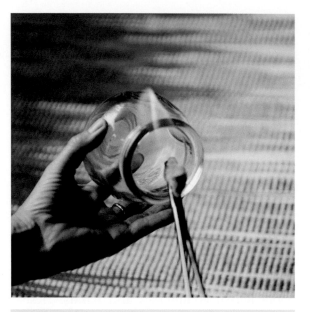

Fig. 21.13
Fire cupping creates suction and space between layers. Traditionally, copper or glass cups are used.

strung, cannot switch off, sweating a lot at night and having scary dreams/night terrors.

Prone

Head massage.

Herbal compresses on neck, shoulders, and back.

Plai oil with repetitive laminar groove ironing technique (spinal nerve protocol).

To release stuck Wind and tightly bound fascia, I used cupping (Fig. 21.13) with slow flash cupping (leaving on for a few minutes and taking off, repeating this many times). I also used sliding cups: while not traditional to Thai massage, this technique is relaxing and calming.

This was the first time I have cupped this client and he was amazed at how much he relaxed and how his tremors completely disappeared after the treatment.

Case Study 10 (1 hour)

Shoulder pain and *stiffness*.

Seated

Herbal compresses on neck, shoulders, and thoracic region of back.

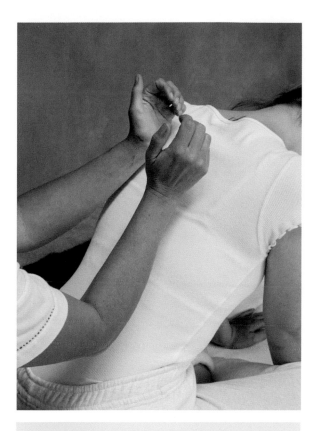

Fig. 21.14
Dtee performed in seated position, with the recipient stabilizing her own position. This is a very traditional posture.

Stretches for neck and shoulders, including forearm rolls.

Deep compressions on shoulders with hands.

Beating (**dtee**; Fig. 21.14).

Khuut.

Range of motion.

Case Study 11 (1.5 hour)

Menstruation pain with clotting and *back-ache.*

Seated

Yoni steam.

Supine

Abdominal massage with compresses and belly oil (see Chapter 22).

Massage down each leg to (and including) feet, with compresses and second layer massage work.

Channel work on legs.

Foot massage.

Lumbar spine traction with scarves (Fig. 21.15).

Case Study 12 (1.5 hours)

Stiff neck and *lower back.* Client enjoys really deep pressure and expressed belief that both areas needed some deep work to relieve the stiffness. This client is generally very *stiff* and *tense*, with really bound-up muscles and not much range of movement.

Prone

Herbal compresses on back, neck, hamstrings, and gluteal muscles.

Forearm rolls.

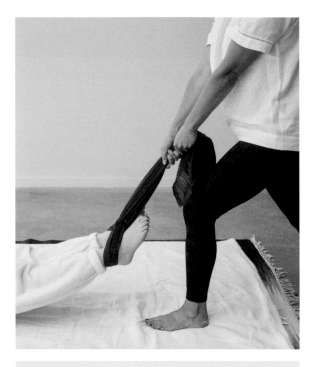

Fig. 21.15
A scarf is tied carefully to provide a stable hold to both legs, so they can be tractioned together.

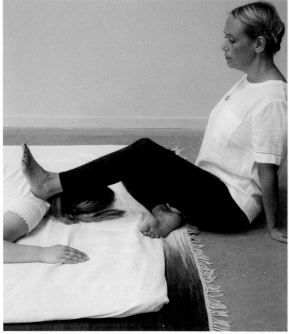

Fig. 21.16
Deep tissue work with the heel is an incredibly effective way of releasing bound-up structures while being very easy on the practitioner's body. The therapist works with melting, slow, and aware touch to ensure safety.

Deep compressions.

Myofascial release stretches.

Heel work in shoulder area (Fig. 21.16).

Lumbar and sacro-iliac joint stretch.

Supine

Compresses on neck while stretching back.

Foot work on hamstrings.

Stretches such as pulling bent leg, gentle knee across leg twist, knee under gluteal muscles each side, big twist both ways.

Golden balm on neck to warm muscles and penetrate the layers.

Foot on shoulder stretch.

Scarf work to massage neck (Fig. 21.17).

Traction with scarf.

Seated

Beating.

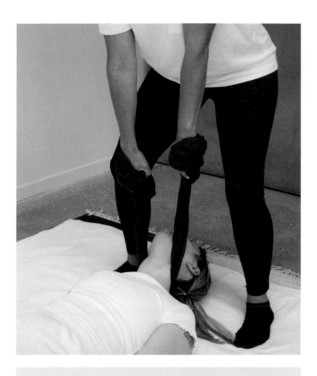

Side note: Disclaimer – some of these techniques need instruction from a teacher and lots of practice before they are safe to use. I do not recommend their use without this instruction and practice, as they can be very harmful.

Fig. 21.17
Skill and instruction are needed to work on the cervical spine with scarves. It is deep bodywork in an area that can be very sensitive and vulnerable.

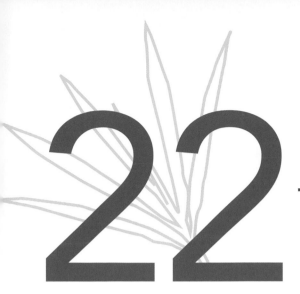

22 Treatment Protocols

In this chapter we look at some effective protocols for working on the neuro-vascular bundles, spinal nerves, and viscera. These are tried and tested, ancient practices that are nevertheless rarely taught or known of in either Western Thai massage or the wider complementary therapy community. They highlight the diversity of therapeutic Thai massage when approached through the original, traditional lens.

Wind Gates

"Wind Gates" are often referred to and taught as "blood stops," which is both dangerous and inaccurate. Words are very important: they resonate, have impact, and are therefore significant. The misuse of this term also indicates that the technique has not been taught with the correct theory behind it, something that is incredibly important for safety reasons. I have known people (myself included) pass out from the "blood-stopping" technique and it is almost impossible to arrange professional insurance if you say you practice it. However, Wind Gates are a different thing all together.

Wind Gates are referred to in Thai as "Bpra Dtoo Lom," which means "opening the Wind Gates."

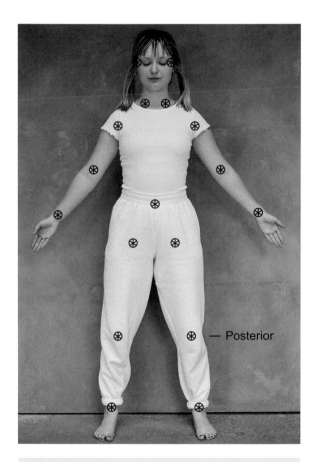

Fig. 22.1
Location of Wind Gates, which correspond to plexuses and give access to many Sên.

Chapter 22

This technique uses a gentle "touch input" that triggers the body to correct itself through work on the neuro-vascular bundles. The pressure of touch is extremely light, as this is the depth needed to feel the arterial pulse. With training, the practitioner can feel the rhythm of the heartbeat and its extended heart tree at these pulses. This is slow work that takes time, precision, and an acute "listening touch." The practitioner must work with focus and attention to be able to recognize the subtle shifts that happen.

As the pulse is *gently* and partially occluded, it will alter, sometimes speeding up, other times slowing down. It can grow stronger or weaker. The practitioner senses its rhythm and quality, and feels it go through a stage of changing (when it can become irregular) before it settles. When it does settle, the work has been done. The practitioner waits for a couple of seconds, holding the pulse and checking it is steady before slowly releasing it.

As the name suggests, when opening the Wind Gates, the practitioner is concentrating on the movement of Wind in *all* of the Sên, as it needs to flow through them all, and not just the arteries.

Location of Wind Gates

The pulses are located at the bends in the body (joints; Fig. 22.1). These are areas where the pulse can be gently engaged near the body surface. The pulse is used as a tool for location, yet it is *all* the Sên that are being stimulated, not only the arteries. This is where the Wind Gates are located:

- foot (pedal artery)
- back of knee (popliteal artery)
- groin (femoral artery)
- navel (descending aorta)
- armpit (axillary pulse)
- elbow (brachial artery)
- wrist (radial artery)
- neck (carotid artery).

How to Work the Wind Gates

Start by palpating to find the pulse. Make sure you are in the right place and then use your body *lightly* to engage the pulse, very gently and not occluding. If you press too hard when feeling for the pulse, you are likely to miss it entirely or occlude the artery in a dangerous and detrimental way.

The navel, axillary, and femoral pulses (Fig. 22.2) are more easily located using the center of the palm of the hand, whereas the others can be located using the flat of the fingers.

I suggest you do this work in a calm and quiet environment where you can concentrate fully and not be distracted. If the recipient tends to be chatty, you can ask them to be quiet for this work. This will help you concentrate and their breathing will relax.

Side note: The level of pressure you use is the weight of your arm without any leaning pressure. This is a light-touch technique. Hold it very steady without moving.

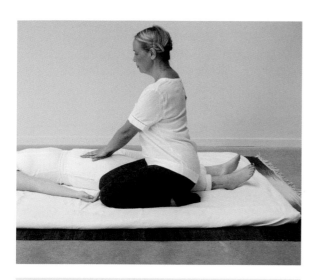

Fig. 22.2
The femoral Wind gate. Wind gates are worked with gentle, concentrated touch, as the changes in pulse are very subtle.

Side note: I once had my axillary pulse occluded (a blood stop), which caused damage to the neuro-vascular bundle (Sên) in my arm. It made my arms feel really heavy, as if they had no blood going to them, and this effect lasted for a number of days.

Indications

Wind Gate treatment is specifically beneficial for balancing the Winds. It can be used in various ways: for example, to enliven or wake up a limb by encouraging a flow of Wind to it, which has a resetting effect.

Wind Gate work can be performed at the beginning of a treatment to help circulation problems or to accommodate a level of sensitivity that makes other, deeper, work difficult. It helps to bring Winds to an area and, with them, the nourishment of fresh blood and nutrients.

It can be used at the end of layer work to correct Wind in the joints. Joints are often problem areas and there can be a build-up of congestion, toxins, and stagnation. Wind Gate work is fantastic for flushing this out and getting it all moving. It tells the pulse to calm and can be helpful for high blood pressure.

Wind Gate work is good when someone is off balance, which will show if they are nervous or on edge, cannot switch off, or are stuck in an unhealthy cycle of thoughts. Subtle Wind Gate work also stabilizes the rhythms of the body, balancing and resetting them. It controls and manages movement in the channels. It is often deeply relaxing, and the recipient may feel a rush of warmth or cold as the Sên are cleared and the Wind rushes through the body, taking fresh blood and nutrients with it.

Wind Gate work can be helpful for all element imbalances due to its balancing of the Winds, which then has an effect on all the other, slower, elements.

Before embarking on Wind Gate work, it is important to care for the layers as follows:

- Work on the skin, tissue, and Sên of the whole area.

- Use vibration and mobilization for the joint on which you intend to do Wind Gate work.

- Work the Wind Gate for that joint.

- Mobilize the joint again.

- Move to the next area.

Cautions

Side note: I do not recommend that this technique be used at all without instruction from a teacher.

Each Wind Gate can be worked on a maximum of three times in a session, but the practitioner should be clear about *why* they are repeating the work, as it is often as effective and sufficient to do it once only.

Work only one Wind Gate at a time, so that all the focus and attention can be on that. Do not split your focus between two areas, as it is likely that the pulses will have different qualities that would be easily missed if working bilaterally.

On slim patients, take extra care when working on the navel Wind Gate. Ensure that it is engaged but the pressure is still light; this will avoid any compression on the descending aorta where there is not much superficial fascia to protect it.

Side note: Navel Wind Gate work should not be carried out during pregnancy.

Side note: As always, if in any doubt, leave it out. Check in with your teacher and discuss so you can be guided.

Spinal Nerve Treatment

This is an excellent example of when the recipient receives treatment directly to the skin with oil. It is a wonderful therapy that can calm, nourish,

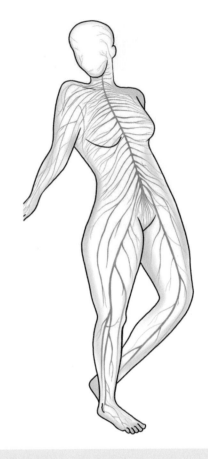

Fig. 22.3
Spinal nerves innervate the whole body and are pathways of movement, called Sên in Thai medicine.

and energize. This is especially useful when the recipient is functioning below par or when they cannot have direct work done on the abdomen.

As the spinal nerve treatment addresses the nerves, it can be used for both physical and emotional issues. Emotionally, it is beneficial when someone is nervous, agitated, on edge, chaotic, Windy and restless, or has insomnia. On a physical level, it is indicated when digestion is painful, sluggish, fast, or unsettled. Working with this protocol is also beneficial when the recipient has numbness, neuralgia, fibromyalgia, sciatica, peripheral neuropathy, or post-stroke or any other condition affecting the nervous system, both sympathetic and parasympathetic. These are Western medical terms, which are not how a Thai medicine practitioner would look at a condition, but they are used here to give an understanding of how Sên can affect the body.

The spinal nerves innervate the whole body, from the head to the feet, and function as motor, sensory, and autonomic pathways between the brain and the entire body (Fig. 22.3). In Thai medicine these pathways are Sên: different names but the same underlying meaning. There are thirty-one pairs of nerves in total, traveling from cervical to thoracic to lumbar to sacral and coccygeal areas. They form an interesting pattern, one that you might be familiar with seeing in the veins on a leaf. The nerves are close neighbors at the cervical spine but as they travel downwards they become less intimate, with wider spaces between them.

Preparation

As with all Thai massage treatment, the layers should be cared for, and the spinal nerve treatment is no exception to this rule.

I ask recipients to take off their top or T-shirt and I use a scarf or towel to cover them. Traditionally, the female recipient would wear a top with an opening at the back, while men can be unclothed on their upper body.

Herbal compresses are brilliant for soothing the recipient and getting medicinal herbs into the skin, tissue, Sên, and bone layers as preparatory work (Fig. 22.4). They can be used

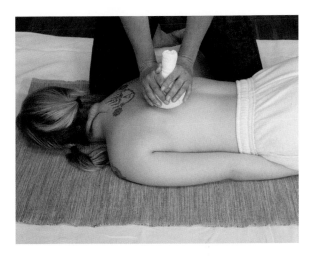

Fig. 22.4
Herbal compresses are used as preparatory tools to open the layers of the body before spinal nerve treatment.

initially through fabric. (If you do not have herbal compresses to hand, you can rub the skin and do some techniques such as rolling, stretching, and deep compressions to address the tissue layer.) The Sên are worked specifically with the nerve treatment.

Oil

There is an herbal recipe for a liniment that specifically addresses the nerves and is the most beneficial when carrying out this treatment; in its absence, it would be a good idea to use *raw* sesame oil, which has warming medicinal properties and is nourishing for Sên.

Spinal Nerve Treatment Protocol

After caring for the skin and tissue with the appropriate tools in your toolkit, you start working directly on the skin.

Chapter 22

Move your body so that you are kneeling or in proposal pose by the recipient's head. Make *all* moves in a downward direction.

1. Put a small amount of oil in the palm of your hand.

2. Rub your hands together and apply oil to the whole back from shoulders to sacrum. You can repeat this to ensure that the oil is evenly distributed.

3. Use your fingers to rub vigorously down the spinal laminar grooves – fingers alternate, not hurrying, to work from cervical spine to sacrum. This means that each inferior and superior move is repeated a few times before the fingers slide a little further down the back and the technique is repeated continuously. The intention is to wake up the nerves by stimulating them.

4. Cross your thumbs so they form a "V," with the right thumb over the left. Place them so that the V is over the spine (Fig. 22.5). Your hands stretch out to achieve as much coverage as possible. Work with thumbs down the laminar groove twenty-one times.

Side note: The laminar groove is found between the spinous process and the transverse process. As muscles soften here, you can reach the tiny transversospinalis muscles on both sides of the spine.

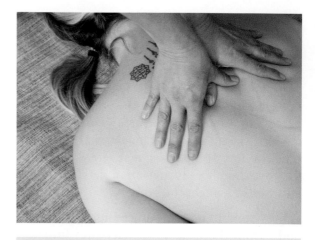

Fig. 22.5
Using thumbs to work into the laminar groove as a technique to release the transversospinalis muscles, which enables tiny nerve fibers also to release.

You can swap your thumbs halfway through the repetitions so that the left thumb is over the right. Your whole hand is active and gliding down the tissue of the back, but the main focus is working the channels with the thumbs.

5. Make your right hand into a fist and place the flat part of your hand, from the knuckles to the first joints of the metacarpals, on the recipient's back (Fig. 22.6a). The line of the first joints will be on the groove on the right side of the recipient's back (from your viewpoint). Place your left hand flat over the bent fingers (Fig. 22.6b). Let the outstretched fingers guide and keep you in place as you slide your knuckles down the groove seven times.

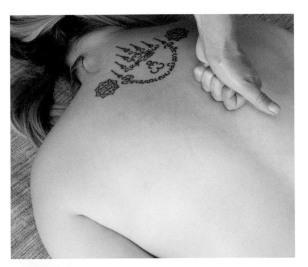

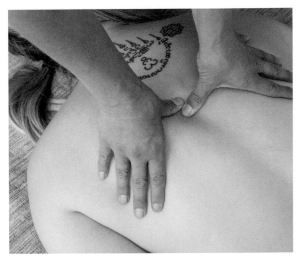

Fig. 22.7
Two thumbs pressing into the laminar groove in an inferior direction.

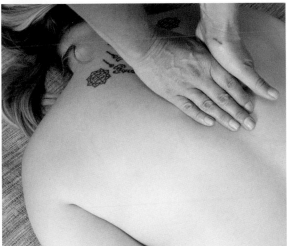

Fig. 22.6
Sliding the knuckles down the laminar groove.
a. Showing the hand position and use of knuckles. b. Showing the hand covering the knuckles and guiding the working hand.

6. Change hands and repeat on the left side.

7. Thumb-press the right side of the groove three times (Fig. 22.7).

8. Thumb-press the left side of the groove three times.

   Move your body so that you are now working from the side of the recipient, in kneeling or proposal pose across their body.

9. Bend your first finger and place it on one side of the spine in the groove. Use the thumb tip of the same hand in the groove on the other side of the spine. Mirror this with your other hand. Press and walk the

tips of your bent finger or thumb down the spine between each vertebra. Keep your arms straight.

Variation: you can also bend both middle and forefingers (left and right hands) and use the joints to press into the spaces between vertebrae.

Move so that you are kneeling near the head.

10. Repeat the "V" thumb slides twenty-one times.

11. Place your right hand on the recipient's left shoulder, and glide your hand to the left shoulder. Place your left hand on the recipient's right shoulder, and glide it to their left shoulder (Fig. 22.8). Repeat, using the right hand going left, and the left hand going right, all the way down the back to smooth it out. Repeat three times.

12. Cover the recipient with a scarf, cloth, or towel.

13. Perform a cross-hand stretch. Place one hand on the recipient's right pelvis and the other hand on the recipient's left shoulder near the scapula. Lean in and stretch the two hands away in opposite directions. Repeat on the other side (Fig. 22.9).

14. Place one hand on the lumbar and one hand across the spine in line with the scapula. Stretch the hands away from each other (Fig. 22.10).

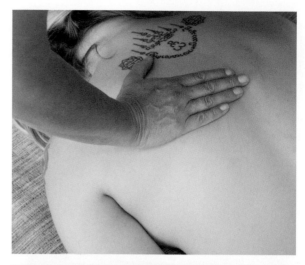

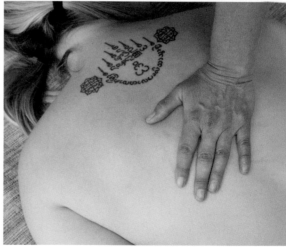

Fig. 22.8
Flat hands sweeping and smoothing out the back right to left (a), then left to right (b).

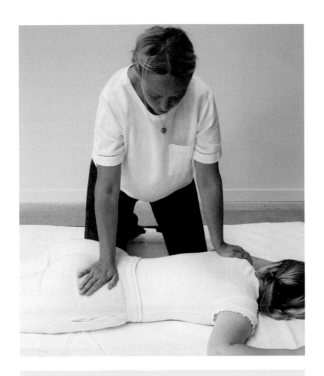

Fig. 22.9
Cross-directional myofascial stretching of the second layer.

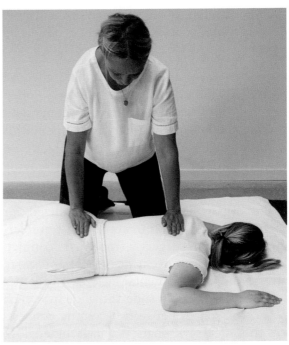

Fig. 22.10
Myofascial stretching directly on the midline.

Abdominal Massage (Nuadt Tawng)

Visceral work on the abdomen and surrounding tissues is vitally important for the health of the whole body, its function, and the emotional core. This area is richly innervated, with an abundance of Sên. Its role as intelligent communicator (also known as the "gut brain") is significant to the entire body, from sensory experience to mental health and vitality (see Chapter 12 for more information).

The massage is concentrated on the organs at the belly, but these are in direct fascial continuity with, and have a close relationship to, the heart and lungs. The Sên (extensions of the heart and nerve trees) are also stimulated within the abdominal massage protocol and so it is important to notice that, as pathways of movement, the three brains (brain, heart, and gut) are being activated and treated as one.

Massage to the abdomen is wonderfully relaxing and assists the recipient in noticing themselves at a very deep level. The experience of receiving Thai abdominal massage is like traveling into the depths of one's body. As each layer is massaged, the recipient's interoception (sense of the internal body) is actuated and there is a feeling of sliding inwards and being fully present in oneself. This work requires the practitioner to be very sensitive, both in the physical hands-on work and in the deeper aspects that are potentially being experienced by the recipient.

Belly massage is one of the most effective treatments for many conditions, often unrelated to the gut. A client may come with limited shoulder movement or neck pain; this may not be resolved by working directly on those areas but often improves from moving the Wind and creating space in the abdomen.

The organs can become immobilized for many reasons: inflammation, food intolerances, injury, surgery, emotional conflict, lack of physical movement or self-expression, stress, and environmental factors. It becomes less easy for them to slide and glide over each other, the spaces between becoming congested. This affects lymphatic drainage, blood flow, and nerve conduction to and from a specific organ, which in turn influences both posture and function. Using manual therapy to create space in this area is the best way to improve and reduce the problem.

How Do I Work on the Belly?

The simple answer is "slowly." It is also important to have had class instruction from a teacher and to know the anatomy of the belly before working on it. More than any other area, the belly needs to be touched and cared for with sensitivity. If you imagine all the internal structures, the vital life-giving and sustaining organs that are housed within the abdomen, it is no surprise that it needs to be treated with respect. This is also where the reproductive organs can be touched on.

As you work your way slowly through the layers, I suggest you imagine *exactly* what

your hands might be touching. While you may not have had the benefit of time in the dissection lab, there is still something very powerful about connecting your thoughts and intention with what your hands are doing and the structures they may be touching. Even if, like me, you have been fortunate enough to explore the inner spaces of the body, be aware that the viscera can be organized in surprising ways. Some organs are not in the place you might think they will be, and there are also congenital presentations such as "situs inversus," where the organs are mirrored to the opposite side. (This is rare, but it is possible for the recipient to have had this condition and yet to have been unaware of it their whole life. I have seen kidneys pushed up and hiding in the ribcage near the lungs.)

The arrangement of the organ layer is unique to the individual and is influenced by functional movement, posture, self-expression, breath, daily habits, and genetics. All of these factors, and many more, can affect the internal organization of any area of the body, including the viscera. This means that the organs are not always located as they may be depicted in anatomical reference literature, so practitioners must be able to identify, through palpation, exactly what structure they are addressing. This work needs guidance from a teacher and experienced, skilled hands to ensure safety and efficacy.

The abdomen is often an area where emotions are stored, and touching this area is likely to bring strong feelings to the surface. Some clients feel self-conscious, while others are not used to having this area touched, especially in a therapeutic environment, and it might make them feel vulnerable or uneasy. If a client has had surgery here, there may be physical and emotional trauma and scar tissue, which can harden and pull internally if not cared for, having far-reaching effects. Others will find being touched in this area *very* soothing and nurturing. Either way, the practitioner needs to approach this work with sensitivity and provide appropriate care for each layer.

I have seen a case where a loved one's belly presented internal bruising in a circular pattern from diaphragm to pelvis after experiencing physical trauma that she tried to emotionally process alone. The bruising baffled the doctors who saw her, but I think that (as it was not abuse) it was her gut visibly expressing pain, alerting both her and her loved ones to the fact that something was seriously amiss.

Massaging the body from the skin to the deepest layers can help to disperse pathogens that reside at the body's core by encouraging it to process toxins more quickly through stimulating optimum function of the internal organs. Adhesions, tightness, pain, lack of movement, constipation, and loose bowels can all be addressed through Thai bodywork techniques that have stood the test of time. In so doing, everything can be freed up and the client is made to feel much more comfortable, with improved posture, a feeling of space and lightness, and increased absorption of nutrients.

Massaging gently and with increased sensitivity is essential around this area. Really tune in to your listening hands so that you can pick up on the subtle shifts that occur, and become intimately aware of the layers. Observe if emotions rise to the surface, detect where there are sore or tender areas, and then work appropriately with the receiver. Keep in mind the physiological and energetic effect you are producing while working around the navel and abdomen, having the intention to encourage change but never forcing it to happen. Patience is the name of the game.

For people who have a lot of energy and cannot calm down, the abdomen is a good place to start a treatment, working through the layers moving fluids and blood out to the extremities. These individuals are presenting agitated Fire element, so you are going straight to the core of the Fire that is burning in them and dispersing it. This will also help slow down the digestion of food so that nutrients can be extracted from it, rather than it moving so quickly through the body that the person becomes depleted (in one end and out the other).

Likewise, someone who is very depleted of energy will respond best to a treatment that brings everything towards the core to nourish it. This will encourage the Fire in their belly to be stimulated. The blood, lymph, and fluids are moved towards the core of the body, where the organs can start to process them. In this instance, massage the abdomen at the end of the session, allowing ample time for the work (as a guide, 30–60 minutes into the treatment).

If someone is really stuck in their head, overthinking, anxious, or worried, I would start with the head and neck and work on the belly at the end, with the intention of working away from their tension to the core for processing of the stress chemicals. In working this way, the treatment starts at the biggest source of the problem and moves to the core.

Most therapists who work with herbal compresses have a passion for them, and never more so than for use on the belly, where they come into their own. The heat and medicinal herbs can do safe, soothing, and deep work, which is especially useful if there is pain and tenderness that does not allow working with the hands. Some sessions could consist entirely of herbal compresses on the abdomen, and I always start abdomen work with them. I have never met a client who does not enjoy having their belly massaged with them.

If you do not have compresses available, then use the technique of rubbing the area to work on the skin, with the intention of bringing blood and heat to the surface. When your hands feel warm from this work and the belly also feels warm, then the skin layer has been cared for.

It is good to palpate the area gently, checking in with the recipient and asking for feedback as you do this. Gently feel your way around, noticing heat, tenderness, and soft and hard areas.

I like to work the front and back of the body at the same time to warm up the whole area with touch. For this I use a technique I named "belly ball," which cares for the skin and tissue layer, and structures in the back of the body, bringing touch input to the erector spinae muscle, kidneys, spleen, and posterior visceral organs.

Indications for Nuadt Tawng

This technique:

- can release deeply stored emotions and toxins

- creates space in the tissues

- moves Wind (making physiological change happen in the whole body)

- addresses hormonal and endocrine imbalances

- replenishes and nourishes the tissues

- influences alignment of the pelvis and organs in situ

- supports organ function

- increases slide and glide so that organs can function at their best

- calms and relaxes

- improves immune function

- addresses essence (vitality of the body)

- improves blood flow and quality

- releases the diaphragm and assists in improving breath

- improves tone

- reduces bloating and indigestion

- improves absorption of nutrients

- relieves pain

- improves posture

- improves pelvic health

- improves menstrual cycles

- encourages healthy emotional connection to the area

- connects heart, gut, and brain.

The practitioner might choose to work on the fifth layer for many reasons. I have listed some, but not all, of these here:

- menstrual or hormonal imbalance

- constipation, diarrhea, reflux

- pelvic misalignment

- back pain

- restricted, shallow breathing

- toxicity and stagnation

- depletion

- low energy/vitality

- poor posture

- being under par, anxious, highly strung.

Contraindications

- Pregnancy.

- Swelling of the organs.

- Crohn's disease.

- Food in stomach.

- Inflammation in whole body (compresses only).

- Kidney stones (compresses only).

General Abdominal Treatment Protocol

The following is a general protocol; it is a good place to start and get some practice, but please note that it is not the complete abdominal treatment, as this should be taught in class by an experienced teacher for guidance.

1. Palpate the abdomen to feel for textural information from the layers, looking for bound-up places and feeling for heat or cold, while initiating touch to the area.

2. Use herbal compresses to warm the area. Either place them directly on the skin or, if they are too hot, on a scarf or piece of cloth placed over the belly (Fig. 22.11). If compresses are not yet part of your toolkit, you can rub the belly to care for the skin or apply warming liniments.

3. Place a small amount of oil in the palm of one hand, rub your hands together, and gently apply the oil to the belly, focusing on the skin layer by massaging superficially. This will build trust and encourage the recipient to start relaxing.

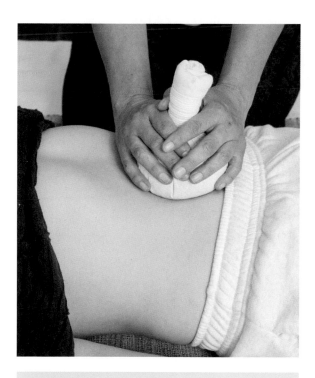

Fig. 22.11
Herbal compresses work on the layers of the belly. A specific traditional formula penetrates to the visceral layer.

4. Work *gently* on the second layer, making sure you are not going deeper than this and concentrating on getting the tissue moving. This layer needs time and the process should not be hurried. There are many techniques that are beneficial, most of which involve pushing and pulling the tissue (Fig. 22.12), dragging it away from bone (ribcage and pelvis), and working into areas of tension with long, slow holds to release them. Alternatively, apply small myofascial stretches to the tissue layer.

Compressions on the abdomen are never as deep as on other areas of the body. Fingers can be used to push or pull away from the midline (Fig. 22.13).

5. *If and when* the second layer has released enough, the channels can be worked. Make sure you do not move on if this area still needs attention. The channels are not deep here but are on the edge of muscles or the central tendinous channel (that is, slightly deeper than the second layer, although you have to "feel" the body you are working on).

There are three channels. The first is the linea alba, the central line from the xyphoid process to the pubic symphysis (a tendinous line on the abdominal wall). Thumb-press the line first with a lateral move, then repeat with a medial move. Thumb-press this channel a third time with an inferior move (Fig. 22.14).

The second and third channels relate to the rectus abdominis on either side of the navel. Both of these are worked medially with thumb presses.

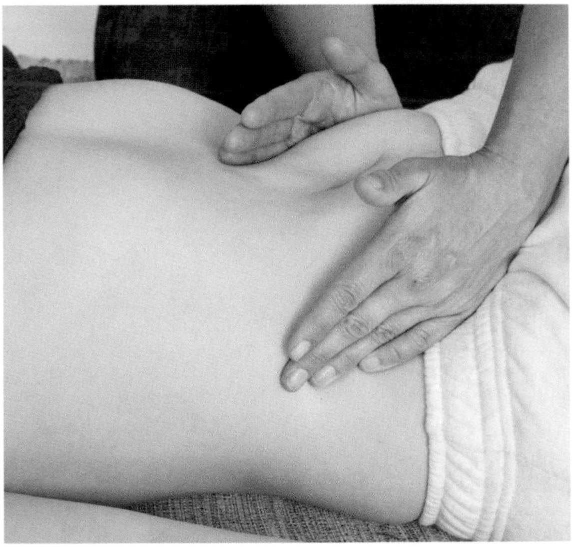

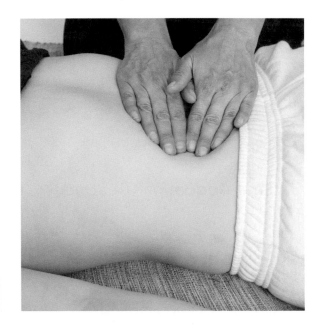

Fig. 22.12
The sides of the hands are used to move the tissue layer.

Fig. 22.13
Fingers are used to work directionally on the tissue layer away from the midline.

The point-specific work for the organs needs to be done with the utmost care and knowledge of the placement of organs and their function. If the recipient finds it intense and you notice they are taking breaths to cope, ease off and ask them to inhale as the pressure is applied, and exhale as it is released (this is the opposite to how most people breath in yoga). The points for the organs are located where the organs are, and the bodywork on organs affects those organs (Fig. 22.15). (There is no distal referral in Thai medical theory.)

Note: the direction of pressure and depth of pressure to each organ are important and instruction should be given by a teacher.

6. Work the points on either side of both inguinal ligament points – inferior above, superior below.

7. For vibration, place the hands (one on top of the other) on the abdomen in various places, making quick presses into the area to shake things up.

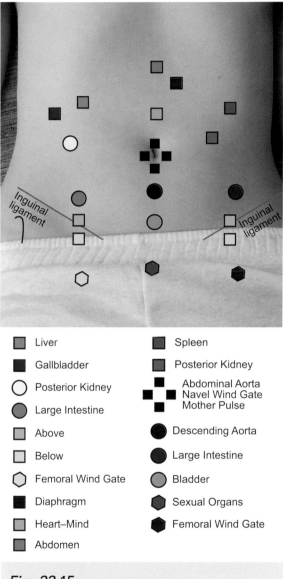

Fig. 22.15
Location of organ points.

▨ Liver	▨ Spleen
◼ Gallbladder	▨ Posterior Kidney
○ Posterior Kidney	◼ Abdominal Aorta
	Navel Wind Gate
● Large Intestine	Mother Pulse
▢ Above	● Descending Aorta
▢ Below	● Large Intestine
⬡ Femoral Wind Gate	● Bladder
◼ Diaphragm	⬡ Sexual Organs
▨ Heart–Mind	⬡ Femoral Wind Gate
▨ Abdomen	

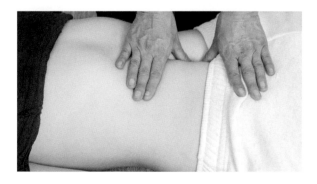

Fig. 22.14
Thumbs pressing into the (linea alba) channel/ Sên.

8. Push up on the abdominal organs with the sides of your hands to lift them, countering the usual movement of gravity and creating space away from the pelvic bowl.

215

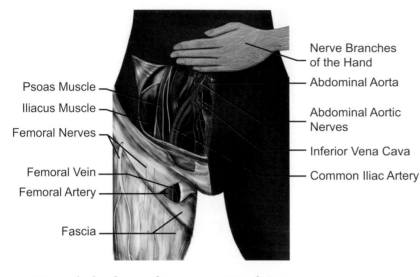

Nerve Branches of the Hand

Psoas Muscle

Iliacus Muscle

Femoral Nerves

Femoral Vein

Femoral Artery

Fascia

Abdominal Aorta

Abdominal Aortic Nerves

Inferior Vena Cava

Common Iliac Artery

Fig. 22.16
The navel Wind Gate and Sên.

9. To work the descending artery Wind Gate, place the center of your palm directly over the navel and sink your hand on to the area, but only until the pulse is felt – no more. This is very light pressure (Fig. 22.16).

10. Work the femoral Wind Gates, one at a time (not bilaterally).

11. Perform three stretches with the legs:

   For the first, bring both of the recipient's knees to their chest and lean your hands on to them. This stretch focuses on squashing the belly.

   For the second, keep the recipient's knees bent and hold them together. Take them first to one side and then the other (the third stretch) to twist the abdominal area.

12. Traction both legs.

13. Scarves can be used at the end of the abdominal treatment. Slide them under the lumbar region of the back and use them to lift the back gently from the floor, giving a gentle back-bend and stimulating the kidneys and spleen (Fig. 22.17).

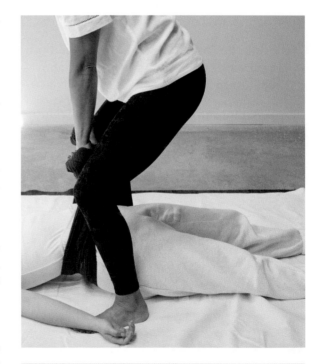

Fig. 22.17
Traditionally, scarves are used as a tool to provide traction and vibration.

23 The Therapeutic Pause

If you have ever had a massage in Thailand, it is very likely that halfway through the treatment, when you relaxed into the deep and intense bodywork experience, the practitioner stood up and walked out of the room, leaving you lying there, wondering if and when they would return. Perhaps they nipped out to use the toilet, but equally they may have gone to make a call or answer the phone, have a chat with their co-worker or family member, or have a snack.

I realize that a break in treatment, while not a deliberate therapeutic factor, does have highly beneficial outcomes. This is because there are times when, for the strongest effect to happen in a treatment, the practitioner must take their hands off and give the recipient's body time to make adjustments and process with no more input. I doubt this is the actual intention of the practitioners in Thailand; it is more likely because there is such a different attitude towards therapeutic medicine, which is seen as practical and part of life with no fuss. This is one of the reasons to think of it more as "kitchen medicine": it does not need anything too elaborate to be effective, and has an everyday simplicity to it without it being ceremonial or complicated.

The space in between manual input is an incredibly therapeutic time where a lot of physiological change can happen. The treatment causes a disruption or release of some kind, and if the body is given time to assimilate this before further work is carried out, it can instigate more change than continuous hands-on work.

This is something I use in my practice. I may walk out of the room during a treatment. I do not want to work with constant physical connection. There is a lot of healing potential in space. The therapeutic pause is an essential part of healing work. It is not following the "I'm doing this to you, I know what's best for you, I am healing or fixing you" model, but instead gives the recipient time to be accepting of themselves in a quiet and restful state. The practitioner can be a catalyst, but it is the recipient's receptivity and the right conditions that create the most change.

In giving a pause to the sensory stimulus activated in a treatment, the central nervous system has time to rest and reset. It is an important part of a treatment, rather than bombarding the body with constant input which can cause inflammation, or overloading the nervous system with too much information.

After a pause, the practitioner can reassess what else, if anything, is needed. Sometimes the area needs more attention, but at other times the practitioner will feel that significant change has taken place, that the therapeutic pause increased this process, and any more work could be counterproductive.

It might feel a bold step to move away, or out of the room, but it is something that an advanced practitioner will have the confidence to do. It shows that they are genuinely and acutely aware of what is best for the recipient. In reassessing and palpating, it will be easy to see if change has occurred and if the work has set the ball rolling for healing. Judging when the therapeutic pause (or pauses) should happen comes from treating many people and from the skill of listening hands.

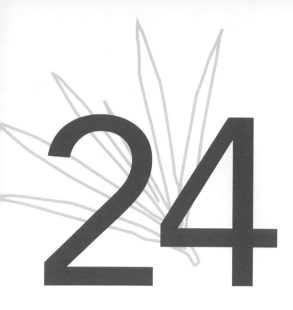

24 Women's Health Care, Pregnancy, and Postpartum

Midwifery is often seen as the sixth root of Thai medicine, yet it is unique in being a tradition preserved purely by women for women. The traditions, knowledge, and wisdom are handed down through the matriarchal line over many generations.

Midwives are traditional doctors specializing in this root, but due to the huge variety of needs a woman has throughout pregnancy and beyond, have extensive knowledge of all five roots. They support women emotionally, psychologically, and physically from conception to the fourth postpartum trimester using herbal formulas, dietary counseling and prescriptions, **Vedic** astrology for diagnosis and spirit medicine practices, and much more, to ensure the health of the mother and baby.

Researching Women's Health Care

In 2017, I traveled to Northern Thailand with a group of women teachers and practitioners who all had a strong interest in women's health. We went there to study and do research with village midwives, using a translator to help us communicate and learn accurately.

We had the most auspicious time, studying in a remote jungle setting and in the homes of our midwife teachers. These women were hugely knowledgeable and generous, pleased to share their wisdom with us. They were able to see that we were all serious about maintaining their traditions and medical knowledge, some of which is now being lost due to modern lifestyles and the younger generations' lack of interest in the ways of the ancestors.

One of our teachers was a midwife living close to the Burmese border, whose father had been a spirit doctor. It was from her matriarchal line that she acquired her knowledge. Her mother, grandmother, and great-grandmother had all delivered babies, and as she sat with us, her teenage daughter joined in to learn alongside us. Our translator was an herbalist and had also delivered babies, as well as having her own. They taught us a lot about the herbs that were growing in their herb garden or were easily foraged from the surrounding landscape (Fig. 24.1). We spent days with them, studying women's practices from their particular tradition, which is from the Chang/Tai people close to Burma. They taught us how to womb-lift, nourish new mothers with medicinal food,

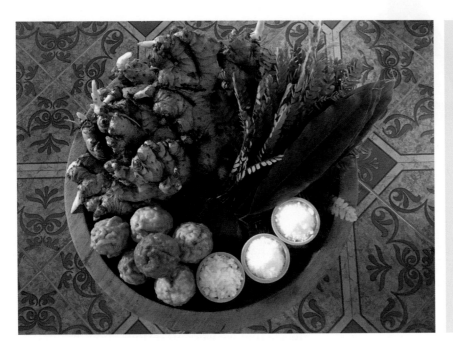

Fig. 24.1
Fresh herbs ready to prepare a general compress.

wrap their bellies, and generally care for them in a way that could be life-changing for future generations and improve the health of so many women around the world.

Studying and researching with these women was a fantastic privilege and very insightful. One of the most remarkable aspects was the level of care a woman would receive after giving birth. There was an acknowledgement of how depleting pregnancy is. For the health of both mother and baby, rest, nourishment, and warmth were *the* remedies. Traditionally and currently in more rural areas, the community supports new parents, bringing food, reciting incantations, making a fire, and keeping it fed twenty-four hours a day for a month, so the new mother can rest in front of it, as well as keeping her company.

We later studied with a Karen teacher who was seventy-five years old and lived in a Shan village. (Karen and Shan are tribes from Northern Thailand.) Her husband had been the village medicine doctor. She too was taught by the women in her family line. There is something very special about the handing down of knowledge through the generations, from woman to woman, mother to daughter, for the education and benefit of the female community. It signifies women's strong connecting force and natural inclination to support each other as they journey through puberty, menarche, pregnancy, birth, miscarriage, and menopause.

We learned huge amounts from these women, and while I would like to research the topic further and write about it in more depth, I also want to impart some of the traditions so that more women can benefit. Some of these traditions are possible to implement in the West, and if they were common practice, they would make a significant difference to women's health.

One of the personal motivators that took me on a research trip of this kind was my own experiences as a woman and mother, and also my observation of a growing need for health care to be very different for the female population. In my practice, I often see long-term, chronic health problems that I recognize as being directly linked to a lack of self-care and education, reproductive issues, pregnancy, and interventions.

The information recorded in this chapter is only a partial representation of the traditional practices, beliefs, and culture that make up this aspect of Thai medicine. Much of this information also comes from time I spent with other teachers in Thailand on the same trip, who shared so generously and patiently with our group as we asked questions and discussed our own personal stories, our shared passion for women's health laying us bare.

Side note: I suggest that any traditional practices involving herbs and heat mentioned in this section are implemented only after sufficient training. While some of them are common in traditions from other parts of the world (and some are undergoing a resurgence, even becoming fashionable), they are written about here in the context of healing practices.

The skin's ability to absorb is used frequently to get herbs into the body, and this is also the case in both general women's health care and postpartum care (and, to a lesser extent, during pregnancy).

In Thai massage and bodywork, medicinal balms, liniments, and compresses are applied to the skin. There are other traditional practices that are specific to women's health, menarche, menopause, and postpartum care.

Side note: The sixth root of Thai medicine is slightly separate and specialized. All other roots are tied into this one, but (unlike the others) midwifery is not interwoven so heavily into the five main roots.

As part of our research, we were taught about many plants, weeds, and herbs that we harvested. We were shown how to implement them using steams, smokes, compresses, and infusions. We were taught the importance of fire, herbal showers, belly binding, internal herbs, and rest.

We then experimented with our own bodies, experiencing for ourselves the effects of each of these wonderful and powerful ancient practices.

Menarche

It is seen as extremely important for women to take extra care of their bodies at the time of their monthly cycle, and doing so is considered to have a beneficial impact on general health for their whole lives. Menstruation is seen as a depleting and cold time, with women's bodies also being more open to spirits. The body is cleansing and detoxifying, the substances being eliminated via the menstrual blood, so in order to support the body, women must keep themselves warm, move a lot, eat nourishing foods, and conserve energy. Additionally, this is a time to avoid cold things such as taking showers and baths, washing the hair, and eating cold foods. Menstruation is a time when a woman may also feel depleted; she may feel low emotionally, have less energy, and feel weak or more tired than normal. These are all signs that her essence or vitality is low.

Pregnancy

Elementally, there is a lot going on during pregnancy. Earth, Water, and Fire elements are all amplified, but these are not seen as imbalances as such. However, pregnancy is seen as a hot condition and anyone who has been pregnant will know this to be true. There is a greater volume of blood running around a woman's body during this time, meaning that she should not use heating herbs, or take saunas or steams. Neither should she take any Wind-increasing herbs, which could cause miscarriage.

Massage in Pregnancy

If working with pregnant women, it is important for appropriate training to be taken to work safely and with confidence.

First trimester

Massage during pregnancy is not advised during the first trimester. You will find this precaution all over the world and it is probably due to this being the time when a woman is most likely to miscarry. It is also the period during which the baby's Kwan (life force) is not yet strong (it takes between six and twelve weeks for it to settle) and could easily be harmed.

Second trimester

While massage *is* possible during pregnancy, it is used only when needed. The second trimester tends to be when the woman has most energy and feels at her best, yet there are huge changes occurring in her body.

The introduction of massage as a relaxing treatment is much more of a Western/contemporary concept. Traditionally, a massage would be carried out for backache, stiffness, swelling, or any other conditions common to pregnancy. The techniques are generally broad-pressured and focus on the skin and tissue layer. Deep work around the legs is to be avoided. Massage is performed in seated or side-lying position.

Traditionally, there would not be lots of stretches performed on a pregnant woman (actually, they tend to stretch less in Thailand generally), and we asked a lot of questions about this. There are large amounts of hormones circulating around a pregnant woman's body that relax ligaments and joints, making stretching ill-advised from both Thai and Western perspectives, especially from the second trimester onwards. Some fascial stretches can be beneficial, perhaps to open up the chest or stretch the neck (these areas also carry the weight of heavy breasts), or to get fluids moving in the ankles, which tend to swell. Herbal compresses are the best way to treat a pregnant woman's body, using floral, gentle, cooling herbs such as peppermint, and other substances like coconut, rice, jasmine, and rose flowers.

Salt is drying and drawing, so should not be added to compresses.

Third trimester

Herbal compresses continue to be a wonderful treatment, given in side-lying and seated positions (Fig. 24.2). With these, you can do some effective work in a short timeframe, an essential consideration as women are often quite uncomfortable. Some *gentle* massage of the abdomen with oil is also helpful at this stage, when skin starts feeling stretched and tight.

Side note: I do not recommend practicing these techniques or using herbs with a pregnant woman unless you have received training with a teacher.

Morning Sickness

Two common medicines are used to help the symptoms of morning sickness: **Ya Hom** (an internal formula) and **Ya Dom** (sniff medicine, similar to an herbal smelling salt) (see Resources).

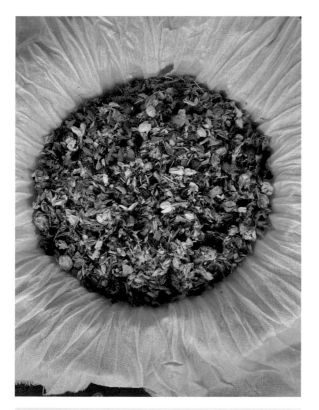

Fig. 24.2
Herbal formula for compresses used in pregnancy, by kind permission of David Crépaud.

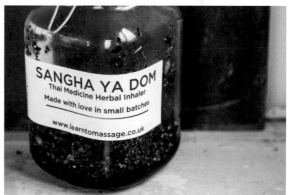

Fig. 24.3
Ya Dom herbal formula is a type of sniff medicine. There are many varieties to be found all over Thailand. This jar is called "Sangha Ya Dom," as it is for communal use.

Gentle massage can be applied to the sternum and front of chest, with the practitioner using palms to rotate away from the midline. This technique should not be applied for too long until after the first trimester.

Womb Lifting

This is a traditional hands-on technique that can be used after six months to ease back and pelvic pain. It creates space for the baby to move more freely and encourages fluids and the fetus away from the lumbar spine and pelvis, where it may be pushing down and pressing on nerves and bone. The technique of lifting up is called **Yok Kwan**. It requires special training and in-depth knowledge of the individual before being applied.

When I was pregnant, my baby was breech with feet first and neck extended (meaning she was also back to front). I used to walk along the street heavily pregnant and have my pelvis kicked by her. This would almost knock me off my feet and I would often have to hold on to something to stop myself falling to the ground. Recalling the sensations I was having in my body back then, I know that Yok Kwan would have felt really good. I remember feeling really weighed down, my back aching and not knowing what I could do about it. Yok Kwan would have created space for my baby to move, perhaps even to a better birthing position.

Birth

Every woman who has ever given birth has had a unique experience. Women love to talk about their birth experiences, despite them ranging from being traumatic and exhausting to empowering – or, conversely, disempowering. They sometimes go according to plan but mostly do not, and in those hours lives and bodies are changed forever.

Nowadays, intervention is the norm, with C-sections and assisted delivery in a hospital environment being far more common than home births. This is also true in Thailand, unless the woman is living in a remote or poor village, but in days gone by, giving birth at home was customary.

Traditionally, a woman would have given birth holding on to a rope suspended above her head and with her husband supporting her body in a seated position from behind. Generally, the woman would be encouraged to do gentle breathing throughout labor, as energy is best conserved for the birth.

Massage in Labor

If a woman has back pain during labor, her back is massaged with the palms of hands in a circling motion, pressing and spreading outwards and downwards.

Postpartum (Fourth Trimester)

Birth is extremely depleting: there are many physiological processes going on, and the amount of energy needed to grow and birth a baby is huge. While pregnancy is a hot condition, the postpartum period is seen as a cold one. Care for women at this stage is paramount to their long-term health: they need all the help they can get to restore their essence. This is vastly overlooked in modern-day culture, especially in the West, where women rush to get back to work. The pressure on women (from themselves as much as society) to "get their bodies back" is immense. Women are really suffering from this, as the need for community and support, rest and warmth, is overlooked to the detriment of women's health.

What stood out for me when I was learning about traditional Thai postpartum care was that women were treated like royalty, with an absolute acknowledgement of the awe-inspiring job their body had just completed – growing and birthing a human. I felt very moved by all that I learned about the traditions of care at the time. First and foremost, for one month, whether the baby was born by natural or C-section delivery, women were given rest, warmth, and nourishment to replenish their depleted essence.

During the postpartum time, there is an increase in Wind element due to water being depleted, and this needs to be nourished by Fire element. The woman is looked after by her husband and the larger community, who will take care of everything so that she can rest in the warmth of the fire (**Yuu Fai**; see later in this chapter). It may seem odd, in a country where it is always hot, that a fire is deemed necessary to nourish and replenish, which shows how great the depletion of a woman's essence is, and how much heat is needed to transform that depletion.

> Side note: Young children are generally kept away from a woman doing Yuu Fai because they are likely to speak the truth about how hot it is, whereas everyone else is playing it down to help the woman cope.

The postpartum woman will not bathe or shower for the month of Yuu Fai but she will wash with warm water infused with herbs from her herbal tea, her skin absorbing them. After birth, the first hair wash and whole-body wash will be with sompoy water (see Chapter 20) with dry or fresh turmeric, which is used for cleaning negative energies, and for protection against spirits and ghosts. She will drink medicinal teas, served warm and made with heating herbs to help nourish and rebuild her essence.

Breastfeeding

Compresses are used to encourage milk production and let-down. They are steam-heated and the breasts, shoulders, upper back, and legs are massaged with them.

Postpartum Practices

Belly binding

After giving birth, the mother needs to wrap her belly tightly with a long cloth. This is done with the intention of supporting the healing of her uterus and other organs, as well as keeping her warm. Wrapping the belly encourages the tissue and organs to return to their natural and healthy position. If the linea alba (the fascial tendinous groove of the midline that runs from the xyphoid process to the pubis) has opened, binding helps it join back together. This cloth also supports the lower back and feels very comforting.

A 6–8-foot (2–2.5-meter) piece of cotton is wrapped very tightly around the area stretching from under the belly up to the diaphragm. This takes a little practice and it is easier if

225

someone else wraps it around for you. The fabric is then tied in place and can be worn under or over clothes.

When I tried out the belly binding, it was incredibly supportive for my back. I did not want to take it off. I noticed that it encouraged me to be more upright. I have also used it since when I have had abdominal pain and bloating, and it was very comforting, the warmth it generated bringing Fire element (heat) to my digestive system to nourish the Wind.

Belly binding can be used after hysterectomy and other surgery, to keep the kidneys warm if someone has depleted essence, and to improve posture. It could also be beneficial for hiatus hernias.

By the fire (Yuu Fai)

It is of the utmost importance that a woman stays warm for one month after giving birth. I say warm, but really it is more like hot. The fire will nourish her and encourage healing at a time that is seen as very depleting. She should lie in front of the fire, with her belly and head wrapped up. During the month of Yuu Fai she should lie on her side, feeding the baby and resting, doing *nothing* else. She needs complete rest and is not allowed to cook, wash, move around, or do anything strenuous. It is a time for replenishing, feeding, and bonding.

In the West, women can either lie in front of an open fire or, if they do not have one, use a device such as a halogen heater. A special recipe uses specific herbs that should be taken if Yuu Fai has not been possible at all:

- ginger
- black pepper
- plumbago
- alum
- acacia.

Clay pot

A clay pot with a lid, containing heated rock salt, is used on the belly and all over to massage the body and help draw out fluids (Fig. 24.4). This helps reduce the massive increase in body fluids from pregnancy, drawing them

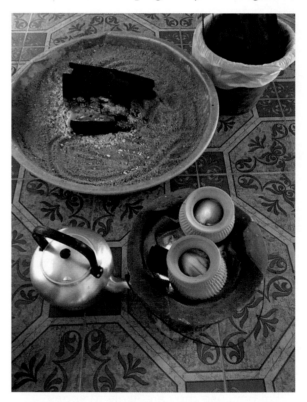

Fig. 24.4
Clay pot with salt and herbs to assist the woman's body to heal after giving birth.

out and eliminating them. Assisting the uterus to contract quickly will prevent infection, stopping it pushing on the bladder and further preventing the potential for incontinence and a weak pelvic floor. A clay pot can be used if the woman is bleeding a lot after giving birth.

After a C-section, the clay pot cannot be used, as the scar needs time to heal.

Yoni steam

The practice of Yoni steaming is incredibly healing and beneficial, and a great way to get herbs into this area of the body. The woman sits over the steaming herbs for a while before receiving an abdominal massage. When I treat my clients, they steam, then have abdominal massage with herbal compresses to break things up and move the stagnation of blood and toxins, and then steam again. This is also a deeply relaxing and soothing treatment, and is highly effective. I have achieved fantastic results with it: for example, one client has been given the all-clear for a cyst that has disappeared; another now has a regular menstrual cycle without pain, having suffered for many years. Yoni steaming can be helpful for the menopause, painful menstruation, dryness, or hormonal imbalances, and for general self-care of the reproductive organs.

Vaginal steams are used postpartum to clear out the uterus and encourage healing. The woman sits on a chair with a hole cut out of it, above a vessel that is full of steaming herbs. The herbs specifically assist healing and cleaning of the uterus and any debris left in the birthing canal after the delivery. They also

improve muscle tone and restore fluids, essential care after labor.

Side note: Yoni steaming is an ancient practice that recently has come under a lot of scrutiny in the Western world. It has been labeled as unsafe and damaging, yet has been used widely throughout many cultures and centuries. However, it should be practiced only when there is a need for it.

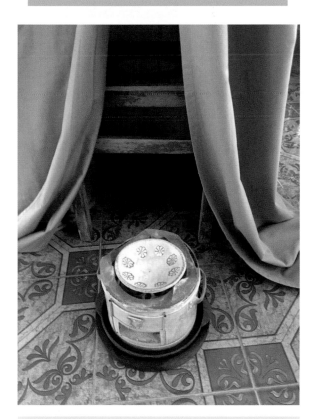

Fig. 24.5
Yoni smoke tent.

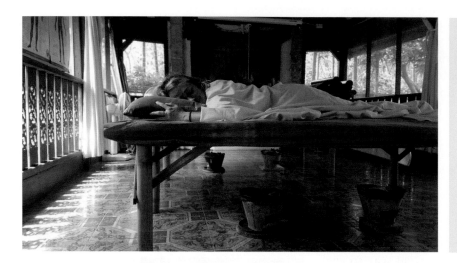

Fig. 24.6
Grilling bed with layers of medicinal herbs to lie on.

Yoni smoke

The Yoni smoke involves lighting a charcoal fire contained in a bucket. A recipe of medicinal herbs is placed in a vessel on the fire, which should be smoldering but not flaming. A chair with a hole cut out of it is positioned above the fire. A one-person tent suspended from the ceiling gives privacy.

The aim of this particular practice is to speed up the retraction of the uterus after giving birth. Smoking helps control postpartum hemorrhage (which naturally happens when the placenta breaks away from the uterine wall) and stops bleeding.

Grilling bed

This not only is for postpartum use, but also helps with stiffness, detoxifying, circulation, and stagnation. It calms the mind and nourishes essence.

A **grilling bed** (Fig. 24.6) consists of a wooden bed with slats and two or three charcoal buckets below. A layer of herbs is placed directly on the bed with a cotton sheet covering it. When the person lies down on it, they also cover themselves in a sheet, lying on their front and back for as long as is comfortable.

Pregnant Massage Practitioners

Traditionally, women would not massage when pregnant, as they are seen as being much more susceptible to harm by particular spirits who like blood and waste products and will cause women to be sick, or during menstruation, as it could exacerbate their depletion and lead to sickness. There are some healing practices that women are not allowed to perform at all, as they are seen to be more open to being harmed by spirits.

If we work in the Western world as massage practitioners, it may not be possible to reschedule a week of clients or take a week off work to rest and conserve energy. However, it is worth keeping in mind that the body is processing, cleansing, and detoxifying during this time, and being more vigilant with nourishing self-care.

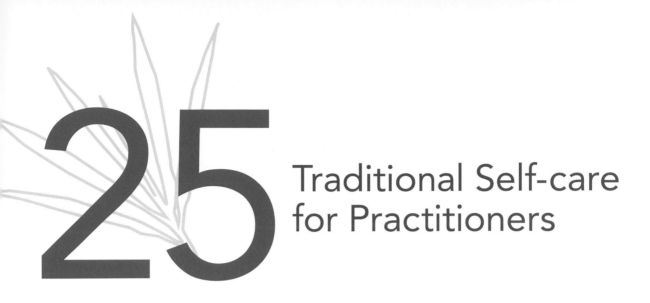

25 Traditional Self-care for Practitioners

The **Wai Kru** is taught at the beginning of a course in Thai medicine study and should be an important part of a practitioner's daily practice.

As you will see, it pays respect to the three main figureheads of Thai Medicine (Buddha, Reusi, and the father doctor **Jivaka Kumarabhacca** – see later), as well as honoring parents and teachers (Fig. 25.1).

There are many variations on Wai Kru and it is traditional to carry out the practice twice a day, morning and evening. The sacred words are meant to be spoken with a deep, resonant voice.

Traditional Wai Kru is written in Pali, an ancient language of Theravada Buddhism. Pali is the Buddhist equivalent to Latin for Catholics.

Wai is a gesture made with the hands, in which the palms are bought together. This communicates respect and is offered as a humble request, or to convey hello, goodbye, and thank you.

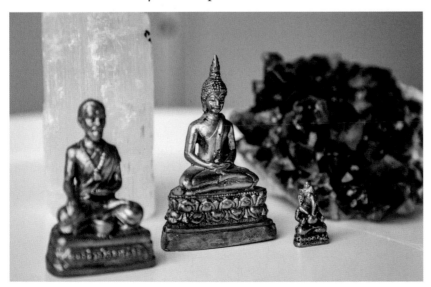

Fig. 25.1
Buddha is honored as the ultimate healer. He has Jivaka on his right and Ganesh on his left. The crystals symbolize Earth element. By kind permission of Katie Bracher.

Chapter 25

Kru translates simply as teacher. You can see from the list below that it is commonplace for there to be a daily practice that gives thanks to teachers. In traditional Thai culture, teachers of the healing arts are seen as being further along the path of enlightenment; they carry on the teachings of the Buddha, are part of a Sangha, and take on the role of being like parents to their students.

General Wai Krus are found in many parts of Thai life. There are many variations that are recited in all walks of life. The healing arts version specifically recognizes parents and teachers.

The Healing Arts Wai Kru

The Wai Kru:

- Pays homage to the Buddha for being the ultimate healer.

- Pays homage to the Buddha Dhamma. These are specifically the teachings of the Buddha, who taught ways to lead a harmonious life and to ease suffering in the world.

- Honors the Sangha (a community that carries on the teaching of the Buddha and any communities that support you personally).

- Pays respect to parents for giving life.

- Pays reverence to current and past teachers for the knowledge they have passed on. It recognizes that wisdom comes from our predecessors and gives thanks for the passed-on knowledge.

- Contains verses for presenting offerings to guides and helpers; these could be spirit guides or any beings who have helped in this or a previous life.

- Includes further verses asking for guidance and protection, which can be called for from teachers, spirits, and ancestors.

- Pays reverence to Mother Earth in the form of a deity called **Mae Thorani** (Fig. 25.2).

- Pays reverence to Ganesh (see Fig. 25.1) and many other deities (that are holders and protectors of the Dhamma), as well as honoring any guides and spirits.

- Acknowledges the father doctor, Jivaka Kumarabhacca, for his compassion to all beings. He is also extremely highly regarded and respected for his service to medicine throughout Asia, which included being a physician to the Buddha, as well as an obstetrician.

- Acknowledges the Reusi of old and of the present day for their dedication and studies of the natural world, and for sharing their knowledge, from which Reusi Dat Ton, herbal medicine, and Thai bodywork developed.

- Includes verses that ask for forgiveness for any intentional or unintentional harm that may have been caused.

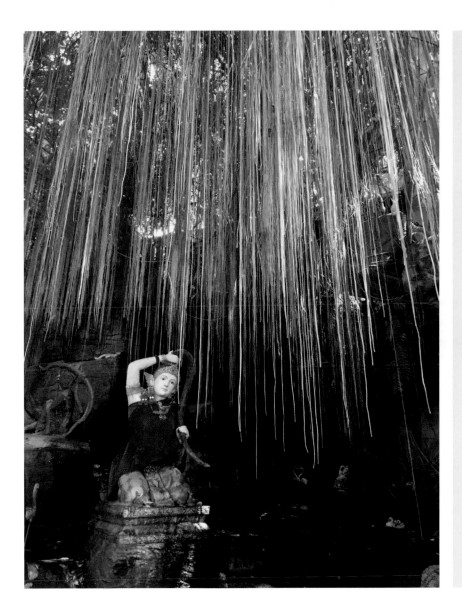

Fig. 25.2
A statue of Mae
Thorani, the Mother
Earth deity, in the
grounds of a temple
in Bangkok.

- Has verses for the Brahmaviharas and the precepts (see next section), and for taking comfort in the Buddha, Dhamma, and Sangha. During the practice, after reciting each Brahmavihara, the practitioner meditates on these qualities for a while to build connection to them, so they can extend those qualities outwards to their communities and beyond.

The Brahmaviharas

- **Metta** – loosely translates as loving kindness to all beings.

- **Karuna** – compassion to all beings, hoping they will be free from loss and suffering.

- **Mudhita** – sharing in the happiness of all beings. Joy, praise, and wealth for all beings.

- **Upekka** – balanced, clear understanding.

The Precepts

The precepts are similar to vows and are a code of ethics for healing arts practitioners. They include:

- not harming and striving to help

- not taking that which is not given, and making the effort to return something to its rightful owner

- not being involved in adultery or sexual misconduct, which causes disharmony in a community

- not being unkind with words, including gossip or false promises

- abstaining from any mind-altering drugs, which make a practitioner unable to help someone in need safely or to make decisions with a clear mind.

Healing Mantra

At the end of a massage, if you want to chant something to clear the physical space of energies or **Lom Pit** (evil Wind) and to cleanse yourself, this **mantra** is very helpful. It can also be recited during cleansing the physical body with Sompoy water. It is repeated three, five, seven, or nine times. It is about resting on Buddha, Dharma, Sangha, and our teachers for support.

Buddham Paccakami

Damman Paccakami

Sangham Paccakami

Gurupajihayacariyam paccakami

Glossary

Access points specific points that are very sensitive to touch and are busy with Sên.

Accessory cells various cells of the immune system that interact with T-lymphocytes in the commencement of the immune response.

Acro-yoga a physical practice that combines yoga and acrobatics.

Amulet a small object worn to ward off evil, harm, or illness, or to bring good fortune.

Andrographis a widely used, bitter-tasting herb with anti-inflammatory, antiviral, and antioxidant properties.

Angulimala an important figure in Buddhism.

Aponeurosis a strong sheet of white fibrous tissue.

Awakeness the state of being awake to oneself.

Ayurvedic a system of medicine with historical roots in India.

Ban a technique that shakes a bony area such as a hand or foot.

Benjagoon one of the oldest Thai medicine herbal formulas.

Bite a term coined for when the pressure or range of stretch is faultless and exact.

Blood-letting a treatment that withdraws blood from a patient/client to cure illness.

Bpao the act of blowing sacred words on to the body.

Bpra Dtoo Lom a term that translates as opening the wind gates.

Brahmaviharas a series of four Buddhist qualities and the meditation practices to cultivate them.

Buddha Dhamma teachings of the Buddha.

Cadaver an embalmed body.

Cancellous denoting bone tissue with a mesh-like structure.

Channels fascial connections between two structures which are pressed to target Sên.

Chet a spirit medicine technique involving a leaf or root.

Chi (qi) invisible energy, life force; from the Chinese medical system and related to meridians.

Chyme partly digested food and gastric juices.

Collagen a protein component of connective tissue which gives elasticity and support. It is found in skin, bones, teeth, ligaments, blood vessels, and tendons.

Core element constitution genetic traits which give information about physical and personality traits and disease predisposition.

Cranio-sacral describes a gentle type of bodywork therapy.

Crus (of the diaphragm) one of two tendinous structures that form a tether for muscular contraction and which extend to the vertebrae.

Cupping an ancient therapy that uses cups applied to the skin to create suction.

Decoction a method of extraction that involves boiling herbal or plant material such as stems, roots, bark, and rhizomes.

Dermal of the skin.

Dermatome a specific area of the skin that is supplied by one spinal nerve root and that transmits information from the skin to the brain.

Din Earth element.

Dtee beating, a technique/percussive therapy.

Edema the medical term for fluid retention in the body.

End-feel tissue resistance to motion, stretching, or pressure at the end of range.

Endoderm one of the three types of primary cells formed in the very early embryo.

Endomysium a thin membrane of fascia surrounding and separating tiny muscle fibers.

Endorphins a group of hormones secreted in the brain.

Enteric refers to a division of the autonomic nervous system that resides in the gastro-intestinal tract.

Epidermal relating to the outermost layer of the skin.

Epimysium the fascial sheath surrounding a muscle.

Erythema a response in the superficial capillaries of the skin which causes redness due to an increase in blood flow.

Fai Fire element.

Fascia an interwoven system of connective tissue with varying textures and functions, found everywhere throughout the body; helps to support and protect muscles and organs, connects body regions, and creates differential movement between layers.

Fire cupping a treatment that uses glass cups on the skin to create suction.

Gaia-Ya-Bam-Bat one of the roots of Thai medicine, known as physical therapy.

Galea aponeurotica a tough fibrous sheath or aponeurosis that forms the middle layer of the scalp.

Geomancy a method of divination that interprets marks on the ground; also known as "Earth divination."

Greater omentum a large, apron-like structure of visceral peritoneum.

Grilling bed a traditional postpartum practice in which a woman lies down on a bed with herbs and heating underneath her.

Grooves fascial connections between two structures that are pressed to stimulate Sên.

Gua Sha an ancient bodywork technique used in Chinese medicine to scrape the skin.

Haek an ancient spirit medicine technique.

Hypodermis a whole-body layer of subcutaneous tissue between the skin and deep fascia, known also as adipose tissue or superficial fascia.

Interoception internal perception or internal sense.

Interstitial situated within a particular organ or tissue.

Jit Jai Thai phrase meaning heart–mind.

Jivaka Kumarabhacca the father of medicine, recognized throughout Asia.

Karma cause and effect from past and present lifetimes.

Karuna the Buddhist quality of "compassion to all beings."

Khuut a technique used to scrape the skin with a tool.

Kinetic describes the energy associated with motion.

Kwan the life-force spirit of the whole body and each individual body part and organ.

Lanna an indigenous people from Northern Thailand.

Linea alba a fibrous tendon on the anterior abdominal wall which connects the xyphoid process of the sternum and the pubic symphysis of the pelvis.

Lom Wind, movement.

Lom Pit poisonous and toxic Wind released from the body during or after scraping and cupping.

Luk Prakhob a traditional Thai treatment using herbal compresses.

Lymph nodes structures that form part of the immune system and which filter substances in the lymphatic fluid.

Mae Thorani the Mother Earth deity.

Mala a set of 108 beads in the form of a necklace, used for meditation, reciting, and chanting.

Mantra words with sacred and spiritual powers, often with one syllable, sound, or word/group of words.

Mechanoreceptors receptors on the skin that detect sensations of touch.

Menarche commencement of menstruation.

Mesentery the tissue by which the visceral organs are attached to the posterior walls of the abdomen by a fold of peritoneum.

Mesoderm one of the layers of cells developed very early in utero.

Metta the Buddhist quality of loving kindness.

Morphology the study of the size, shape, and structure of biological and anatomical things.

Mudhita the Buddhist quality of vicarious joy.

Myelin a sheath of fascia around nerves which insulates and enables the movement of electrical impulses throughout the central nervous system (brain and spinal cord).

Myofascial describes a type of connective tissue/fascia in the body.

Myotome a group of muscles that are supplied by one spinal nerve root.

Naharu broken Sên, such as nerves or veins.

Nam Water element.

Nociception perception of a neural signal produced by specialized sensory receptors in the peripheral nervous system.

Nociceptors sensory pain receptors that respond to potential threat signals.

Nuadt Tawng the Thai name for abdominal massage.

Glossary

Numerology a divinatory science relating to a number and a coinciding event.

Pali the sacred language of the oldest form of Theravada Buddhism.

Palmistry the study of the palm of the hand to decipher future and past events, elements, and planetary alignment.

Palpation the process of using the hands to assess the body, to ascertain where work is needed.

Parasympathetic describes the part of the autonomic nervous system related to resting and repair.

Parkinson's disease a condition that affects the brain, causing shaking and stiffening of the muscles.

Perifascia a thin membrane of fascia allowing for deferential movement.

Peristaltic describes muscular contractions of the digestive tract.

Peritoneum a serous membrane lining the abdominal wall and encapsulating visceral organs.

Piezo electric relates to the storage of energy within fascia and bone.

Piriformis a deep rotator muscle in the buttock area.

Plai a medicinal rhizome root found in many Thai formulas (English name Casumunar ginger).

Pleura a serous membrane that envelops the lungs and covers the thoracic cavity, which houses the lungs, heart, and thymus.

Plucking a technique that specifically works on Sên.

Proprioception awareness of the position and movement of one's own body.

Proprioceptors sensory receptors that respond to position and movement.

Pulses sites where the artery can be gently compressed near the skin surface and the heartbeat can be palpated by trained fingertips.

Reflected a term used in dissection that means exposed or uncovered.

Release points specific pain points located in the tissue layer on channels that can be worked on to provide release from blockages.

Reusi Thai Buddhist spiritual ascetics or shamans.

Reusi Dat Ton (Reusi, spiritual ascetic; Dat, to stretch; Ton, oneself) an ancient self-care system combining breathwork, stretching, self-massage, chanting, and meditation.

Rishi the Indian counterpart to Thai Reusi.

Rolfing a form of manual therapy originally developed by Ida Rolf.

Sak Yan a spirit medicine tattoo consisting of geometrical, animal, and deity designs, based on Vedic astrology readings.

Sangha a Buddhist monastic order, traditionally composed of four groups: monks, nuns, laymen, and laywomen; often used to describe a community.

Sarcomeres units of striated muscle.

Scalpel a small but extremely sharp bladed instrument, used for surgery and anatomical dissection.

Sên a pathway of movement in the body.

Sên Sumana the abdominal aorta, considered a primary pathway of movement.

Serous fluid one of various body fluids resembling serum.

Serous membrane a thin membrane of fascia that lines the abdominal cavity and other internal organs.

Shaman a practitioner who interacts with the spirit world.

Somanaut an explorer of inner space and the internal structures of the human body.

Somatic relating to the body, as separate from the mind.

Somatosensory system a means of communicating information about the body to the brain via separate receptors and pathways.

Sompoy Acacia seed pods used for tool cleaning and cleansing spirits.

Sternocleidomastoid a muscle that connects the base of the skull to the clavicle and sternum. It flexes and rotates the head, and the vagus nerve lies deep to it.

Suttas ancient texts found in Buddhism.

Symbiotic involving interaction between two different organisms living in close physical association.

Synovial fluid a fluid found in the cavities of synovial joints, which reduces friction during movement.

Tachycardia a condition in which your heart beats more than 100 times per minute.

Tantra an esoteric Buddhist tradition, practice, and technique.

Tarot the study and use of symbolic cards to ascertain information.

Taste systems ways of categorizing herbs, depending on factors such as internal/external application.

Tentorium cerebelli an extension of the dura mater that separates the cerebellum from the inferior portion of the occipital lobes.

Thenar eminence the group of muscles on the palm of the human hand at the base of the thumb.

Theravada the oldest form of Buddhism.

Thermoreceptors specialized nerve cells that are able to detect differences in temperature.

Tok Sên an ancient spirit medicine tool and technique.

Touch receptors sensory neurons located in the skin that possess specialized endings that respond to mechanical stimulation.

Tourette's syndrome a condition that causes a person to make involuntary sounds and movements called tics.

Upekka the Buddhist quality of equanimity.

Vagus nerve the longest of the twelve cranial nerves; often known as the wandering nerve, as it travels from the brain

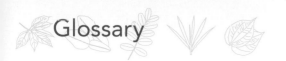

through the thorax and then meanders down to the internal organs.

Vãta the Pali word for Wind.

Vedic refers to the Vedic philosophy of the Hindu religion.

Villi found in the intestine, these structures absorb nutrients from food and move them to the bloodstream.

Viññāna translated as "consciousness," "life force," "mind," or "discernment".

Viscera the internal organs, especially those in the abdominal cavity.

Wai Kru a daily spiritual practice in which students pay respect to the Buddha, their teachers, and their parents, and which formalizes the student–teacher relationship.

Wind Gate a natural junction in the body where Wind is obstructed.

Ya any medicine that is taken internally or externally.

Ya Dom a herbal formula inhaler used for dizziness, sickness, anxiety, insomnia, and respiratory conditions.

Ya Hom an ingested herbal formula for dizziness, sickness, nausea, blocked nose, and vertigo.

Yan a spirit medicine pattern.

Yogi a practitioner of yoga or meditation.

Yok Kwan a hands-on technique to help ease pain during pregnancy; also called "womb lifting."

Yoni a Sanskrit word that indicates the womb and female sexual organs.

Yuu Fai a traditional women's health practice, translated as "staying by the fire" during the postpartum period.

References

Aristotle, 2011. *The Philosophy of Aristotle*. UK: Signet Classic.

Avison, Joanne, 2015. *Yoga, Fascia, Anatomy and Movement*. UK: Handspring.

Concise Oxford English Dictionary, 7th edn, 1988. UK: Oxford University Press.

Finando, Donna, 2005. *Trigger Point Therapy for Myofascial Pain*, 2nd edn. Canada: Healing Arts Press.

Hargrove, Todd, 2014. *A Guide to Better Movement*. USA: Better Movement.

Juhan, Deane, 2003. *Jobs Body: A Handbook for Bodywork*, 3rd edn. USA: Station Hill.

Koch, Liz, 2012. *The Psoas Book*, 3rd edn. USA: Guinea Pig.

Lawton, Gregory T., 2001. "Comparison of somatosensory effects of therapeutic vs. medical massage." *Massage Today* (April).

Lawton, Gregory T., 2009. "A comparison of the somatosensory effects of therapeutic vs. medical massage, Part II." *Massage Today*, available at www.massagetoday.com.

Miller, Jill, 2014. *The Roll Model*. USA: Victory Belt.

Myers, Thomas, 2009. *Anatomy Trains*, 2nd edn. China: Churchill Livingstone/Elsevier.

Oschman, James L., 2000. *Energy Medicine: The Scientific Basis*. USA: Churchill Livingstone.

Pert, Candace, 1999. *The Molecules of Emotion*, 2nd edn. UK: Simon and Schuster.

Turchaninov, Ross, 2000. "Research & massage therapy: Part 1. The science to back it up." Originally published in *Massage Bodywork* (October/November). Available at https://www.massagetherapy.com/articles/.

Wohlleben, Peter, 2017. *The Hidden Life of Trees*. UK: William Collins.

Resources

Thai Massage Training

London Institute of Thai Yoga Massage, UK, Europe and internationally

Danko La Radic, Serbia

Lise Flora Waugh, Pacific Northwest, USA

Nephyr Jacobsen, Oregon, USA

Reusi Dat Ton

David Wells, USA

Ya Dom

Can be purchased by emailing info@learntomassage.co.uk.

Online integral anatomy

Gil Hedley, www.gilhedley.com

Dissection

Julian Baker, www.functionalfascia.com

Gil Hedley, www.gilhedley.com

Practitioners

Natasha De Grunwald, www.natashadegrunwald.com, UK, Europe and internationally

London Institute of Thai Yoga Massage, UK, Europe and internationally

Further reading

Anatomy

Deane Juhan, 2003. *Jobs Body: A Handbook for Bodywork*, 3rd edn. USA: Station Hill.

Liz Koch, 2012. *The Psoas Book*, 3rd edn. USA: Guinea Pig.

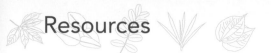
Reusi Dat Ton and Thai Yoga

David Wells, 2016. *Reusi Dat Ton, Part 1: Self Massage and Joint Mobilization of Traditional Thai Yoga.* USA: CreateSpace Independent Publishing Platform, North Charleston, SC.

Thai Medicine and Herbal Formulas

Nephyr Jacobsen, 2015. *Seven Peppercorns.* UK: Findhorn Press.

Pierce Salguero and Nephyr Jacobsen, 2003–13. *Thai Herbal Medicine.* UK: Findhorn Press.

Fig. 7.1   With kind permission of David Wells.

Fig. 7.2   With kind permission of Tim Bewer.

Fig. 8.1   By special permission of Functional Fascia.

Fig. 8.2   By kind permission of Functional Fascia.

Fig. 10.2   With kind permission of Functional Fascia.

Fig. 12.1   By special permission of Functional Fascia.

Fig. 16.1   By special permission of Tim Bewer.

Fig. 16.2   By special permission of Pierce Salguero.

Fig. 16.3   By special permission of Masaru Emoto.

Fig. 16.4   By special permission of Masaru Emoto.

Fig. 16.5   By special permission of Masaru Emoto.

Fig. 19.17 With kind permission of David Wells.

Fig. 21.3   With kind permission of Katie Bracher.

Fig. 24.2   With kind permission of David Crépaud.

Fig. 25.1   With kind permission of Katie Bracher.

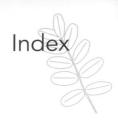

Index

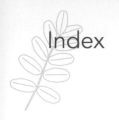

Index

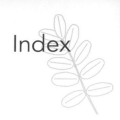

Index